The 90-Minute
BABY SLEEP
Program

Follow Your Child's Natural Sleep Rhythms
for Better Nights and Naps

POLLY MOORE, PH.D.

WORKMAN PUBLISHING • NEW YORK

DEDICATED TO MY CHILDREN, MADDIE AND MAX;
TO MY SISTERS AND BROTHERS,
ALISON AND EMILY AND ROB AND PETE;
AND IN MEMORY OF MY PARENTS,
THERESE AND ROBERT MOORE

● ✳ ●

Library of Congress Cataloging-in-Publication Data is available.
ISBN-13: 978-0-7611-4311-6

Cover and book design by Janet Vicario
Cover and interior photograph © Ruth Jenkinson / Getty Images
Author photo by Philip DeFalco
Charts on pages 10, 12, and 28 adapted from charts by Katherine Sharkey

Workman books are available at special discounts when purchased in bulk for premiums and sales promotions as well as for fundraising or educational use. Special editions or book excerpts can also be created to specification. For details, contact the Special Sales Director at the address below.

WORKMAN PUBLISHING COMPANY
225 Varick Street
New York, NY 10014-4381
Printed in China
First printing January 2008
10 9 8 7 6 5 4 3 2

About the Author

Dr. Polly Moore is the Director of Sleep Research at California Clinical Trials in San Diego. Since receiving her Ph.D. in neuroscience from UCLA, she has worked at the UCSD Cancer Center as well as at the Scripps Clinic Sleep Center, where she researched the effects of sleep rhythms on cancer and pain. She has taught and lectured on the N.A.P.S. plan throughout the United States. She lives in San Diego with her family.

Acknowledgments

To Pam Nagata, coordinator of The Parent Connection, a parenting support group in San Diego County sponsored by Scripps Memorial Hospitals, thank you. Years ago, Pam encouraged me to speak to new parents about infant sleep. Working with these moms and dads has been extremely rewarding. It also helped me develop the material that ultimately formed the core of this book.

To all the moms and dads who've worked with me, especially Amy Harris, Robyn Firtel, David John, Sherry Schnell and Mary Morrow, thank you for your time and attention, and for your insightful questions, your openness, and your willingness to let me know what worked and what didn't.

To Vivian Glyck, thank you for your pivotal encouragement and assistance, including introducing me to Inkwell Management. To Alexis Hurley, Kim Witherspoon, and everyone else at Inkwell, for all your hard work with this project, thank you.

To Kylie Foxx McDonald, Jennifer Griffin, Suzie Bolotin, and the wonderful crew at Workman Publishing, thank you for your guiding words, high standards, and ongoing faith in this book. You've made it a stronger and more useful guide.

To Lynne Lamberg, author of some of my very favorite books about sleep, thank you for your early suggestions on my book proposal, and for your kind support and sage advice along the way.

To Leigh Ann Hirschman, I "literally" owe you more than words can say. For your clarity of thought, fluidity of style, and your passion to make this book better than I realized it could be, thank you. Every single thing you did made it better.

To my gracious bosses and wonderful coworkers at California Clinical Trials, who generously permitted me to work part time while I pursued my dream of writing this book, thank you, all of you.

To all the friends and family who have encouraged me in this project for the better part of the last decade, thank you, thank you, thank you. To those who read and commented on numerous drafts, including Emily Kellndorfer, Ron Szymusiak, Judi Profant Johnson, Gina Poe, Carl Stepnowsky, Sarah Hernandez, and Alison John, I am in your debt. Thank you.

To my beautiful amazing children, Max and Maddie, now seven and nine years old, who've occasionally been heard to grumble as they go off to bed, "Why do I have to have a mom who's a sleep researcher?" I may owe you two the greatest debt of all. Since the day each of you was born, I've hoped to become worthy of the gift and privilege of being your mother. You've taught me so much, you've inspired me, and I simply adore both of you. Thank you. Love, Mom.

Author's Note: *Many parents have generously shared their experiences with the N.A.P.S. plan for this book. To protect their privacy and for the sake of clarity, some of the case studies in this book are composites of those parents' stories. I have been careful to make sure each case study is a fair and faithful representation of the problems families encounter and the solutions they discover when managing their babies' sleep.*

Contents

FOREWORD

If you're an expectant parent or the parent of an infant, you know what it means to worry about your child's sleep. What if the baby doesn't sleep enough? What if he cries all the time? What do I do if the baby won't nap during the day, or if I can't get him to sleep at night? If any of these anxieties sound familiar, you're not alone. Many adults find babies' sleep habits perplexing. Often parents don't know whether a child's fussing means he needs to be fed or changed, whether he's lonely or frightened, or worse, if he's sick or in pain. But an infant's mysterious and "difficult" behaviors, such as irritability and crying, are usually less confounding than they seem.

In *The 90-Minute Baby Sleep Program,* Dr. Polly Moore provides a clear explanation for why infants often fuss—lack of adequate sleep—and a unique and effective program that helps parents improve their baby's sleep *naturally.* Dr. Moore's plan, appropriately titled N.A.P.S., shows parents how to follow one of their baby's natural body clocks (the Basic Rest and Activity Cycle, or BRAC) to facilitate naps and nighttime sleep and maximize a baby's overall sleep time. Her use of the BRAC is a breakthrough: The BRAC is scientifically proven to govern human alertness cycles, and to my knowledge, Dr. Moore is the first to engineer a baby sleep program based on it. And from the glowing reviews of Moore's many clients, it's clear the N.A.P.S. plan really works. It works because it's rooted in science, but also because it's straightforward and easy-to-follow—a boon when you're an exhausted parent up at night with a very tired, very unhappy baby.

I first became acquainted with Dr. Moore some years ago at the Scripps Clinic Sleep Center. The two of us were part of a group of clinicians and researchers who worked together on a variety of sleep research projects. Dr. Moore's extensive experience gives her a unique scope of understanding about how and why the brain sleeps, from the level of the single brain cell to the level of clinic patients with sleep disorders. Her curiosity about the sleep process and her enthusiasm for improving sleep to benefit all patients is infectious, and this was fully apparent to me when I heard Dr. Moore give her talk for new parents. I was most impressed by the way she distilled complex academic research into concrete, accessible advice for parents and caregivers. She achieves the very same feat in this book.

Dr. Moore knows what it feels like to struggle with an infant's sleep. She is not only a neuroscientist and a sleep researcher, she's also the mother of two young children. In fact, she first tested and fine-tuned the N.A.P.S. plan in her own home "laboratory" (the nursery), and found that her children slept better and more consistently once she helped them follow their own inner sleep rhythms.

Whether you co-sleep or want your child to sleep independently, *The 90-Minute Baby Sleep Program* and its N.A.P.S. plan will help both you and your baby sleep better. By putting your baby to bed when she's naturally primed for rest, you'll give her the sleep she needs for cognitive development and emotional growth. And *you'll* rest easier knowing that you're establishing sound sleep habits that will benefit your child through the toddler years, into adolescence, and beyond.

Farhad Shadan, M.D., Ph.D.
Diplomate of the American
Board of Sleep Medicine

Scripps Clinic Sleep Center
La Jolla, California

An Important Note About Sleep Safety

The American Academy of Pediatrics strongly recommends that babies be placed on their backs to sleep. This practice reduces the risk of sudden infant death syndrome (or SIDS, also known as "crib death").

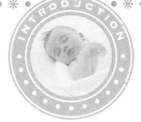

More Sleep, Less Stress

All living creatures—including human beings, dogs, elephants, fish, insects, and even amoebas—are designed to follow natural cycles of rest and activity. Until the widespread use of electric lighting in the late nineteenth century, most humans experienced their rest and activity cycles naturally, going to bed when darkness fell and waking with the sun. Babies and children were permitted to nap when they felt sleepy, and they were allowed to remain asleep as long as necessary.

Today, however, technological advances and our packed daily agendas have led us to live out of phase with our natural rhythms. Sleep has become something we squeeze into the time that's left after pre-dawn commutes and late-night laundry. Over the last several decades, as we've pushed ourselves to work harder and play longer on less sleep, we've demanded that our babies, too, conform to artificial schedules. In the hustle and bustle of life, we've lost sight of two simple facts: how much sleep our babies need, and how to help our babies get it.

Yet sleep is one of your baby's most important jobs in the first year of life, and helping your baby sleep is one of *your* most important jobs as a parent. When you give your baby's sleep needs top priority, you give him a head start on cognitive development and emotional intelligence. Good sleep will help your baby grow strong, with plenty of energy for conquering the world. Without sufficient sleep, our babies suffer, and we parents don't function optimally either.

Luckily, contemporary parents can take advantage of a growing body of knowledge about the internal clocks that govern sleep and waking. This book and its N.A.P.S. plan, which is for expectant parents and for parents of babies up to one year of age (and, to a lesser extent, for toddlers), will show you how to follow one of your baby's natural body clocks. This clock is present from birth and goes strong through the first year, and it helps your baby become sleepy at predictable times. Once you know how to look for these sleep rhythms, you can let them guide your baby into sleeping deeply, soundly, and for longer periods of time, preparing him to master the lifelong art of good sleep. (Note: If your baby is nine months, ten months, or even closing in on his first birthday, you may wonder if this book is worth your time. It is. Within days or even hours after starting the program, you'll see an improvement in your baby's sleep. Better still, you will set the stage for better sleep habits in the toddler years just ahead.)

My Story

I've written this book for you—whether you are a parent-to-be who's heard the horror stories about sleep deprivation or a new parent wondering how you can improve your child's sleep—because I've been there myself. When I was pregnant with my first child, I never expected that my baby would have trouble sleeping. That's because sleep has been my life-long interest and the focus of my career. In childhood, I was fascinated by dreams; in high school, I was curious about my bouts of insomnia (as I later learned, this problem was caused by predictable changes in an adolescent's biological clock). In college and then while pursuing a doctorate in neuroscience, I studied in more detail the devastating results of sleep loss as well as sleep's delicate interaction with psychiatric states and medical illnesses, including cancer. As a neuroscientist focusing on sleep research and disorders, I've spent years working in sleep clinics and academic institutions; nearly every day of my working life has been devoted to the premise that good sleep makes life better. I've seen how inadequate or interrupted sleep has consequences for almost every aspect of a person's life.

So as a scientist, a woman, and a mother-to-be, I was dedicated to good sleep habits. How could I, with my years of specialized training, have trouble getting my baby to sleep? In school I'd been taught that a baby's sleep starts to organize itself after a few weeks and that most babies are sleeping six hours at a stretch by the time they are six weeks old. The textbooks say that by four months, most are sleeping all the way through the night. "It won't be an easy few months," I thought, "but I can handle it." Besides, there were other worries, including breastfeeding and finding child care, competing for my attention as an expectant parent.

Did I have a surprise coming! When my baby, Maddie, arrived, I found that my fancy training did not help me one bit. Sometimes Maddie seemed to want to nurse for astoundingly long and frequent periods; other times she seemed to want a pacifier; sometimes she wanted to be held for hours on end; sometimes she wailed inconsolably and I simply couldn't figure out how to help her. I had steeled myself for disruption and crazy hours and crying, but I had hoped that at least I would be able to interpret my baby's needs and meet them. Even as the months went on and Maddie moved from the newborn phase, I had difficulty telling when she might need to nap or fall asleep in the evening. At night, Maddie would some-times sleep for eight hours at a stretch; other nights were much harder, and as a scientist it bothered me that I didn't know why. Like many par-ents, I developed a set of superstitions about what helped my baby sleep. "The pom-pom worm soothes her to sleep," I'd think, or, "she sleeps better with Mozart playing on the stereo." Then I'd be disappointed when those strategies failed to work on subsequent days.

I consulted with pediatricians, experienced parents, and infant-sleep books. "Newborn babies sleep at random," the experts shrugged. Other parents counseled me not to worry about when or how much my baby slept. "Babies know how to get all the sleep they need," they said. It struck me as odd that no one had anything more concrete to tell new parents.

Because of this advice, I didn't even think to look for a pattern in my baby's sleep. I just kept on going, month after month, thrilled with my daughter but also struggling to make it through each long day and night. Then one morning, when Maddie was about three and a half months old, I noticed that she looked tired and ready for a nap. This surprised me because she'd awakened from a relatively long period of night sleep less than two hours earlier. I didn't expect her to be ready for a nap yet. I remembered that Maddie had shown similar behavior before, and I began to think about this. I looked at the clock, recalled the time that Maddie had awakened in the morning (about 90 minutes earlier), and realized that Maddie's fatigue corresponded with a well-known biological rhythm called the basic rest and activity cycle, or the BRAC. I'd studied the BRAC in graduate school but had never considered applying it to infant sleep.

Had anyone else? I looked at the research. There are many high-quality studies on the BRAC as it relates to several human phenomena, and its foremost researcher had tracked it in his own infant's cycles of wakefulness and sleep. The logical connections between the two were irresistibly strong. At the time, however, this information was literally academic to me. In the informal laboratory of Maddie's nursery—the only lab that really mattered to me at the time—it became clear to me that my daughter showed a distinct and regular biological sleep rhythm. She was not, as I'd been told, sleepy at random times. She became fatigued on a highly predictable basis.

Knowing when my baby was going to be sleepy made other aspects of my life more manageable. When I used my new knowledge of Maddie's sleep rhythms to identify the times that she was ready for sleep, I found that nap times and bedtimes were more predictable and less stressful for both of us. Because Maddie was getting more of the sleep she needed, when she needed it, the mysterious, inconsolable fussiness vanished almost overnight. Her naps were longer, and her nights were greatly improved, with fewer wakings. Although there remained times when Maddie cried (after all, she was still a baby), she was much happier—and I felt that I understood her cries and her needs more clearly.

Other people were able to spot the rhythm in my baby as well. This was true of my brother-in-law, Kevin, who had always felt that babies somehow didn't like him. It seemed to him that every time he tried to hold a baby, the baby started to cry. He would then sheepishly return the child to her parents. When Maddie came along, Kevin wanted to help me out, but he was worried that he wouldn't be able to take good care of her. If you're expecting your first child, you may have similar worries about your lack of experience. But when I taught Kevin about Maddie's sleep rhythm, he felt for the first time that he had a useful guide to infant behavior. He appreciated knowing when she was going to become sleepy, how to interpret the signs of fatigue correctly, and how to take action when those signs appeared. He was no longer afraid or mystified when she cried. Suddenly, Uncle Kevin loved being a babysitter!

It was Kevin and other relatives who insisted that I share my knowledge with other parents. I was skeptical that my services were needed. After all, I wasn't the person who discovered the BRAC, and I wasn't the first to notice its presence in babies. Surely other sleep experts were making this information available to parents already. I nevertheless called a local hospital and asked about participating in their popular lecture series. The director begged me to send a proposal right away. "Sleep is the number one problem for new parents, and many pediatricians don't feel comfortable talking about it." In fact, she explained, pediatricians had stopped giving talks there because the vast majority of questions from parents were about sleep problems in babies, and the doctors felt they didn't have the answers. It turns out that most pediatricians receive very little training in infant sleep problems.

When I gave my first talk, I discovered that other parents were just as hungry as I had been for practical information that would help their babies sleep. Parents also appreciated learning some simple facts about the benefits of sleep, how the sleeping brain regulates itself, and how knowledge of sleep states offers solutions to common problems, such as a sleeping baby's inability to transition from your arms to his crib without waking.

Since then, I've developed the N.A.P.S. plan, a program that's easy for sleep-deprived parents to follow, and I've continued to talk and lecture throughout California and around the United States. The response has been incredible. When I took an informal survey of parents who've attended my classes, eighty-five percent of those responding reported that their babies began to sleep more hours and more regularly when they followed my advice. A significant number were distressed mothers whose babies had been sleeping no more than an hour or two at a time, day and night—an all-too-common phenomenon. A week or so after starting my program, their babies started to nap well and sleep through the night. These parents found the N.A.P.S. plan to be gentle, effective, and easy to implement.

As a mother, I understand that no sleep program will work if it asks you to act against your instincts. My plan can be tailored to your parenting style and to your baby's personality. You can use it and co-sleep if you choose, or you can have your baby sleep in a bassinet or crib. If you want your baby to learn to fall asleep independently at an appropriate age, the N.A.P.S. plan can help you there too. It can also correct a variety of sleep problems in infants up to one year of age. These include:

- Resistance to falling asleep
- Frequent night wakings
- Day/night confusion
- Short naps
- Unpredictable naps
- Difficulty sleeping anywhere other than in a car seat, swing, stroller, or your arms

When you follow your baby's natural rhythms, your child will sleep more and fuss less. When awake, he'll be more content, alert, and playful. You can be confident in knowing that your baby's sleep needs are being met. If you're a first-time parent, that confidence can mark a turning point, as you go from feeling overwhelmed and maybe a little frantic to discovering that you're calmer and more comfortable in your new role. And as you'll learn in the coming chapters, sleep—and plenty of it—is important for the development of a baby's body and brain. The N.A.P.S. plan will not only make you and your baby happier, it will allow your baby to get the deep slumber necessary for a lifetime of good health.

It's easier than you might think to help your baby get restorative and more predictable sleep. Let's get started.

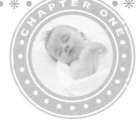

CHAPTER ONE

Sleep, Not Stimulation
A New View

Who doesn't love a sleeping baby? The sight of a baby, swaddled in a soft blanket, cheeks slightly flushed with sleep, touches us deeply. The baby's complete surrender to sleep reminds us of human vulnerability and tenderness. Our innermost desires to nurture and provide are aroused. In the presence of such innocence, we feel both humbled and strengthened by our duty as adult protectors.

As individuals, we appreciate a baby's sleep, but as a culture, we're having trouble getting our babies to sleep well. Sleep difficulties in children are at an all-time high. My experience with new parents strongly suggests widespread, chronic sleep deprivation in babies. Parents who come to my classes describe babies who sleep only twelve or even ten hours a day (far short of the recommended time, which is around sixteen or more hours daily for newborns; see chart below and on page 12. Other parents have babies who spend hours sobbing in their arms before finally nodding off for a short, restless nap. I see babies rubbing their eyes on their mothers' shoulders—even rubbing their eyes on the carpet if they're lying on the floor—while the exhausted parent shakes a brightly colored toy in front of the child and explains, "My baby never seems sleepy!" Many of these parents are unaware that their children are sleep deprived.

In 2005, the National Sleep Foundation (NSF) commissioned a nationwide survey of the sleep habits and behaviors of children younger than four years old. Sleep needs vary across the first year, but according to the NSF's pediatric task force, most babies past the newborn stage need somewhere between thirteen and fifteen hours of sleep in a 24-hour period. And that's just a minimum. Some babies thrive on sixteen hours per day, or even more. But according to the NSF study, about half of the nation's babies log only twelve hours or fewer daily. That's a serious problem: A six-month-old baby who sleeps twelve hours a day will suffer a cumulative sleep loss of hundreds of hours by the end of his first year of life! The study also showed that although parents wish their kids could get more sleep, these parents don't realize their kids actually *need* to sleep more.

Baby's Sleep Distribution*

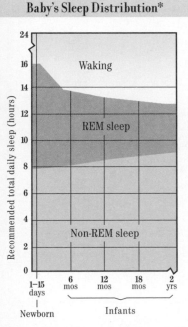

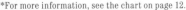

*For more information, see the chart on page 12.

A Sleep-Deprived Generation

Why are our babies missing out on so much sleep? Do parents want to deprive their children of a basic biological need?

Of course not. Like the generations of parents before us, we want to give our babies everything they need and then some. As expectant parents, we may try even harder than our own parents did to prepare for our new job: We take classes or read books about breastfeeding, childproofing, infant cardiopulmonary resuscitation (CPR), and making baby food at home. Yet there are few opportunities to educate ourselves about an infant's sleep. As a society, we tend to assume sleep will take care of itself—or, at least, that there's little we can do to encourage good sleep in our babies or to prevent sleep problems from starting. There's also a widespread belief that the only way to help a baby sleep is to wait until she is six months old and then let her "cry it out" until she learns to sleep on her own and through the night. Many parents are uncomfortable with this approach, not to mention that the six-month milestone can seem awfully distant when your ten-week-old is taking only a few catnaps a day and wakes every hour at night. In fact, there are several steps—most of them very gentle—you can take to promote good sleep habits. It's great if you can start from birth, but you can also implement these steps anytime in the first year to improve your baby's sleep. That's what this book is all about.

But all the sleep science in the world won't make a difference in your baby's sleep habits unless you are committed to helping your baby get the best sleep possible. My program isn't hard to follow, but if you want good results, you'll have to make your child's sleep a priority. For starters, you may need to change your own attitudes toward sleep. Unfortunately, mild sleep deprivation is a way of life for many of us; according to a 2002 NSF study, American adults sleep an average of just 6.9 hours nightly. That's down from nine hours at the beginning at the twentieth century. We are cavalier about our own sleep needs, and some of us may even brag about how little sleep we get at night. In this way, we are poor role models for our children.

Lifetime Sleep Distribution

The recommended sleep averages presented in this chart and the chart on page 10 are intended to help you determine whether your baby needs more sleep than he or she is getting. The figures are culled from the 1966 study cited below, and although they differ slightly from those currently recommended by the National Sleep Foundation, I believe they more accurately reflect the true biological sleep need of babies. The numbers came from observations of actual babies conducted in the mid-1960s, when it was culturally acceptable to let your child nap/sleep as often and as long as necessary.

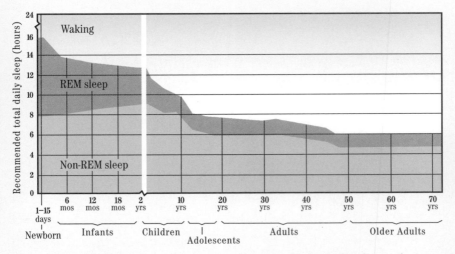

Roffwarg HP, Muzio JN, Dement WC: Ontogenetic development of the human sleep-dream cycle. *Science* (1966); 152:604–619

Even if you have always tried to get sufficient sleep yourself, you probably experience plenty of social pressure to keep your baby awake. In a culture that downplays the importance of sleep for adults, the attitude toward babies' sleep is affected as well. One mother I know recalls excusing herself and her nine-month-old from a playgroup so the baby could take a morning nap. "*My* baby gave up *her* morning nap months ago," crowed another parent in the group. "She's too bright and curious to lie down and go to sleep in the middle of the day." The mother of the napping baby told me, "It made me feel like my child was less intelligent because she needed to sleep." Another mother talks about how the parents in her neighborhood laugh when she puts her baby down for sleep at 7 o'clock in the evening: "When I was growing up, all the kids, not just the babies, went to bed early. Now people think you're a rigid control freak if you don't let your baby stay up late and go out with you to restaurants and friends' houses." On popular television shows, babies don't change the lives of the adult characters; instead, they are simply integrated into their parents' social schedules as cute companions. The message is clear: Sleep is for the slow, the unhip, and the old-fashioned.

WE ARE CAVALIER ABOUT OUR OWN SLEEP NEEDS, AND SOME OF US MAY EVEN BRAG ABOUT HOW LITTLE SLEEP WE GET AT NIGHT. IN THIS WAY, WE ARE POOR ROLE MODELS FOR OUR CHILDREN.

In general, we've fallen for the belief that activity is more important than sleep, no matter what a person's age. Activity—and *only* activity—is supposedly what makes us smart, productive, and fully engaged with life. In the last decade or so, many parents have been taught that babies in particular need constant stimulation if their growing brains are to be properly developed. New mothers and fathers feel compelled to add several items to their to-do lists: Engage the baby with toys that blink, whir, and whistle; take the baby to "Mommy and Me" music, yoga, or other classes; watch so-called educational television shows or DVDs with the baby; and so much more.

Taking care of an infant is a joy. It is also one of the most physically and mentally demanding jobs a person can undertake. Parents nevertheless push themselves to achieve all the items on their list because they believe that the more stimulation they provide, the more effectively they will promote their baby's brain development.

Let's look at the evidence for stimulation and the ability to improve cognitive development. Much of this evidence comes from studies on laboratory rats. Up until the 1960s, it was standard practice for lab rats to be placed three to a cage, with no toys or objects to explore. Then it was discovered that when researchers added two or three additional rat "friends," along with five or six toys, such as wheels or ladders, the rats developed brains with nerve cells that had a more complex pattern of connections. This finding was a huge breakthrough for neuroscience because it showed for the first time that brains can change in response to their environment.

Although all of us—babies and children and parents and grandparents—need challenges and changes to keep our brains growing, it's important not to exaggerate these findings. Many people—including the folks at companies that manufacture infant toys—have interpreted these and other studies to mean that developing brains need a continual bombardment of colors, music, and extravagant playthings. Let's remember that the rats were given a few friends and a couple of sturdy toys to share. We're not talking about a rat Disneyland here. It's vital to have some colorful, safe toys for your baby and to provide stimulation by holding her, playing with her, and talking and singing to her. But we have no proof that structured activities, specialized toys, DVDs, or flashcards lead to improved cognition or better school performance down the road. In fact, too much stimulation can have the opposite effect because it can cut into crucial sleep time for your baby.

Sleeping Brain, Active Brain

The misperception that sleep is a sign of laziness or weakness is understandable. Sleep looks and feels an awful lot like a state we enter when we're too tired to continue our productive work and need to shut down. When we sleep, we are relatively still, and our faces tend to adopt a slack, unthinking expression. Our ability to perceive the world—

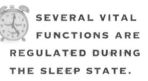 **SEVERAL VITAL FUNCTIONS ARE REGULATED DURING THE SLEEP STATE.**

to hear, feel, and see—is compromised. But in this quiet phase, the body and brain aren't taking a vacation, not at all. Although at present no one can say exactly *why* we sleep, it's clear that several vital functions are regulated during the sleep state. We know this because of the grave consequences of missing out on sleep. A 2006 Institute of Medicine report stated that sleep deprivation in adults is linked to an increased risk of hypertension, diabetes, obesity, depression, heart attack, and stroke. Scientists at the University of Chicago have shown that after just eleven days of sleep restriction, healthy young men develop prediabetic symptoms and produce lower levels of human growth hormone. Other scientists are investigating a connection between sleep loss and poor immune function.

And it's during sleep that the brain has an opportunity for some of its most efficient work. The brain processes information during sleep. It uses sleep time to encode and consolidate what we learned during the day, which may be why our minds feel so sharp and uncluttered after a good night's rest. It's as if all the information from the day has been filed away in its proper place, where it can be retrieved and used to its best purpose. Without sleep, the brain is more like a messy desk full of teetering stacks of papers—it's harder to remember where the most important information is, much less apply that information at the right time.

In a 2002 study of sleep and learning by Harvard researchers Robert Stickgold and Matthew Walker, right-handed students were taught to use their left hands to tap out a complex series of numbers on a keyboard. After a training session, the students increased their speed at the task by about 60 percent. But were they able to improve their performance any further? When the group was tested later that day, the students did not show any improvement. But after going home for a good night's sleep and returning the next morning, the students' speed increased by another 20 percent—even though they had not practiced at all. These and several other findings suggest it's not just stimulation that's important for learning, it's the sleep we get *after* stimulation. These studies also offer a reason why babies sleep so many hours out of each day. According to Dr. Walker, "Their intensity of learning may drive the brain's hunger for large amounts of sleep."

Sleep may also help babies develop abstract thinking, one of the highest levels of thought. In a study at the University of Arizona, researchers played a recording of short phrases from an artificial language to a group of fifteen-month-olds. The language was built on word relationships that are similar to those

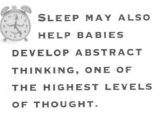 **SLEEP MAY ALSO HELP BABIES DEVELOP ABSTRACT THINKING, ONE OF THE HIGHEST LEVELS OF THOUGHT.**

in English. They played the phrases repeatedly until the babies grew familiar with the sounds. Afterward, some of the babies took naps at their regular times; the others were not scheduled for naps and stayed awake. Four hours later, the researchers played the recordings again. They also played new recordings, using the same artificial language but with new relationships between the first and last words in each phrase. Using a well-established technique for studying infants, the scientists tracked the babies' ability to recognize the sounds by carefully examining their gaze. Both groups of babies were able to recognize the familiar recording—but the babies who had taken naps were better able to take their knowledge of the first recording and use it to help them recognize new patterns in the second.

One of the most compelling arguments for sleep and its connection to learning is a very simple one: It's harder to pay attention or even to care about new information when we're tired. Neuroimaging studies show that the brain has to recruit additional resources and is less efficient when it's sleepy. Tired people are less vigilant, less flexible in their thinking, and less able to solve complex problems, probably because they suffer from apathy toward the task at hand. You've probably had the experience of losing items when you're tired—a classic sign of attention loss—or feeling that you need to summon up reserves of energy just to get simple tasks done. And under those circumstances, who learns well or enjoys life? Although no one has studied the consequences of sleep loss on a baby's attention span directly, I've seen far too many sleep-deprived babies who are unable to focus their attention and take an interest in their world. Sleep helps your baby take more pleasure in her time awake and engage with her environment.

> **SLEEP HELPS YOUR BABY TAKE MORE PLEASURE IN HER TIME AWAKE AND ENGAGE WITH HER ENVIRONMENT.**

Your baby's first year is a critical period when learning occurs at a faster rate than at any other time of life. New babies must learn how to control their limbs, decipher sounds and sights, identify significant people, take in nourishment, and eventually communicate with others and manipulate their surroundings. This is a time when, yes, you want to provide your baby with a loving and reasonably stimulating environment—*and* when you should let her get all the sleep she can, so her developing brain can sort through new information and file away memories of what she's recently learned.

More Sleep Means Less Fussing

There are other reasons to encourage a baby's sleep. One of them is that sleep reduces the mysterious fussing and wailing that send new parents into a panic. Why do babies cry when they're sleepy? Think of it this way. Most of us adults know what it feels like to be sleep deprived. We become irritable, short tempered, impatient, and jumpy. Our tempers are quick to flare and our tears to flow. As the sleepiness accumulates, we may experience the paradox of being so tired we cannot sleep, and it becomes increasingly difficult to calm ourselves.

In this respect, babies are a lot like us. When tired, babies are tearful, edgy, and harder to engage. I've seen many chronically tired babies mislabeled as temperamentally "fussy," "high need," "clingy," or "difficult." Without a well-rested baby for comparison, parents don't realize their babies would be sweeter, more playful, and more fun if they simply had some sleep. Parents may come to expect and tolerate their child's problematic behavior, not realizing they are perpetuating a situation that can be easily reversed with proper sleep management. I once worked with a couple whose eleven-month-old child was difficult to deal with on a frequent, daily basis. They had long ago come to regard her as cranky by nature. Once they followed my instructions, the child began sleeping solidly and for longer periods of time. When awake, she was calmer and more flexible. The difference was so dramatic that the child's father jokingly asked his wife, "Do we have a different daughter?" No, just one who was finally getting the sleep she needed.

Furthermore, it's hard on everyone when a baby is chronically irritable. A baby's seemingly endless fussiness can stress the bond between parents and child. A Canadian study of nearly five hundred mothers showed that moms score lower on vitality tests when their babies rarely seem content and have no regular sleep or feeding times. When mothers are able to predict when their babies will become sleepy, they are less stressed and have more energy to enjoy their babies.

As well-rested babies grow into kids who understand how to sleep well, they have a better chance of developing the emotional control that is linked to sufficient sleep. Kids who get enough sleep are more likely to control their impulses, develop empathy, learn the consequences of their actions, and comfort themselves. It's much harder to set limits with sleep-deprived babies who grow into sleep-deprived big kids. These kids aren't bad kids by nature; instead, they are too tired to control their emotions or focus their attention.

Good Sleep Now Leads to Good Sleep Later

Think back to a more carefree time in your life when you could stay up late on weeknights and then crash for a deliciously long nap on Saturday afternoon. You were taking advantage of your freedom, as well as your body's ability to recover from sleep deprivation. When adults deprive themselves of rest, they can usually compensate with recovery sleep, in which the slow-wave restorative sleep stages are especially deep.

Babies can't do this. Their brains just aren't capable of recovery sleep yet. Just as visual systems, language, and emotional skills are still being formed in the first year of life, a baby's system of sleep regulation is also under construction. In other words, their brains have to *learn* how to sleep. Babies aren't born knowing what it means to feel sleepy, how to fall asleep, how to stay asleep, or how and when to wake up. When babies are allowed all the

WHEN BABIES ARE ALLOWED ALL THE SLEEP THEY NEED, EVENTUALLY THEY LEARN WHAT GOOD SLEEP FEELS LIKE—AND THEY'RE MORE LIKELY TO SLEEP WELL AS OLDER CHILDREN AND ADULTS.

sleep they need, eventually they learn what good sleep feels like—and they're more likely to sleep well as older children and adults.

If sleep loss goes on for long periods of time, babies start to act like nursing home or intensive care patients, who suffer from alertness that feels more like sleep and sleep that's less satisfying. The line between sleeping and waking becomes fuzzy. These babies have poor-quality shallow sleep and are easily awakened. They are also more likely to fight and cry at bedtime because they can't tell when they're sleepy—and because they don't get a positive bounce in the morning from having slept well. Sadly, these babies are at risk for growing into sleep-deprived children and adolescents. You might hear that your baby will simply "grow out of" her sleep problem, but several studies have shown that unresolved sleep problems tend to last well into childhood and perhaps beyond.

That's a scenario you really want to avoid, because there are strong links between sleep loss and serious childhood problems such as attention-deficit/hyperactivity disorder, weight gain, frequent injury and illness, and even growth problems. Sleep loss is also strongly connected with a child's ability to do well in school. A 2005 study in the journal *Sleep* shows that when children are sleep deprived, their teachers are much more likely to describe them as forgetful, inattentive, and slower to understand new information. As kids get older, the stakes get higher: Preadolescents with sleep problems are more likely to be held back at the end of the school year. Well-rested children, however, are at an advantage. Study after study shows that kids who sleep well get higher grades and score higher on cognitive tests. In fact, being well rested is a primary predictor of good school performance. No matter what your educational background, family situation, income, or social status, good sleep is an academic edge you can give your child.

Take a Stand for Sleep

Whenever you feel the pressure to skip your baby's naps in favor of supposedly educational experiences, remember this: The whole world is new to your baby, and she gets plenty of education just by looking at her hands, hearing your voice, playing with safe and simple toys or household objects, or smelling dinner as it cooks.

 SLEEP HELPS A BABY UNDERSTAND WHAT NEW EXPERIENCES MEAN TO HER AND THEN CONVERT THIS UNDERSTANDING INTO PERMANENT LEARNING.

What your baby's brain needs is sleep, and as much sleep as possible, to process this information, remember it, and integrate it with what she already knows. Sleep helps a baby understand what these new experiences mean to her and then convert this understanding into permanent learning. She doesn't need more stimulation in the form of gimmicks or classes, especially if these experiences deprive her of slumber or if they distract you from perceiving signs that she is sleepy.

Now you've got plenty of reasons to stand strong against the cultural pressures that downplay sleep and its importance. Next, let's look at a baby's sleep rhythms and how you can use them to improve your child's sleep.

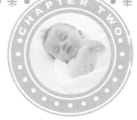
The Beat Goes On
Natural 90-Minute Rhythms

People who are seriously sleep deprived sometimes start to wonder if sleep is truly necessary. After all, they reason, if sleep is a basic biological urge, why are they still upright, walking around and talking and doing their jobs? Why don't they simply crash at their desks after spending the whole night at the office or find themselves lulled into a nap while riding the bus home?

The answer is tucked deep within the brain, in a cluster of nerve cells called the suprachiasmatic nucleus, or SCN. The SCN is the storage facility for the body's clocks. These clocks regulate nearly all of our biological functions and appear in virtually all organisms. Different clocks run different aspects of our physiology. We have clocks that repeat once a year, once a month, once a day, and at other intervals. For example, more babies are born in late summer than at any other time of year, suggesting annual clocks that drive the release of sex hormones. There

DIFFERENT CLOCKS RUN DIFFERENT ASPECTS OF OUR PHYSIOLOGY.

are monthly clocks that regulate a woman's menstrual cycle and ovulation. There are also daily clocks,

known as circadian rhythms, the most famous of which runs an adult's sleep/wake cycle.

The circadian rhythms encourage the release of certain stress hormones—adrenaline, vasopressin, and cortisol—to wake us up in the morning light. (It's no coincidence that the SCN receives direct input from the eye and retina.) As darkness falls, another hormone, melatonin, is released and helps withdraw alertness and prepare us for sleep. Even when we're very tired, after eight hours on the night shift or up all night with a fussy baby, it's hard for us adults to override our circadian rhythms and fully make up for lost night sleep during the day, when we are programmed, as it were, for wakefulness. This is especially true in the morning when the SCN is sending us strong signals to remain alert. Social and environmental cues, such as mealtimes and sunshine, are also powerful contributors to daytime wakefulness. It's the SCN's job to promote wakefulness during the sunlit hours. That's why it's possible to be extremely sleep deprived and still remain awake at your desk or in the nursery.

Aside from daily clocks like the circadian cycle and other yearly and monthly cycles, we have clocks that run for less than a day. These are called ultradian cycles, and they are the key to understanding your baby's sleep.

In the 1950s, sleep research pioneer Nathaniel Kleitman and colleagues discovered that sleep consists of two distinct states: rapid eye movement (REM), the sleep state in which dreams take place, and non-rapid eye movement (NREM). These two states are strikingly different. REM sleep is quite active. It's so active, in fact, that sleep researchers often call it "paradoxical sleep": The paradox is a highly active brain associated with a fully resting body. During REM, electrical signals in the brain's cortex (the gray matter cap on the outer surface of the brain, recognizable by its folds and creases) are intense, firing in irregular patterns similar to the ones that occur during wakeful periods. Visual imagery and dreams occur in REM, and your breathing and heart rates are uneven. Your muscles may twitch, and brief facial expressions—a grimace, a faint smile—may flit across your face. In this state, your brain uses almost as much energy as it does during waking. When allowed to wake up naturally, without the aid of an alarm clock or a wailing baby, we most often do so at the end of an REM sleep cycle, possibly because of REM's similarity to the waking state.

In contrast, NREM sleep is the restful power-off state that most people associate with deep sleep. In NREM, your body is generally immobile; even your eyes are still. You may experience some dream-like activity, but it does not resemble the vivid, imagistic, and narrative dreams associated with REM. Your heart rate and respiration slow down, becoming more regular and even. Although brain activity continues in NREM, it is very different. Electrical signals throughout the cortex become more synchronized and regular, and large groups of nerve cells begin to fire in a simultaneous rhythm. Compare the nerve cells in the cortex to a stadium full of people: When you're in REM sleep, people all over the stadium are having little snippets of excited conversation among themselves. It's a wildly active, creative time. When you begin NREM sleep, it's as if these smaller conversations quiet down as people turn their attention toward the game. Soon large groups of people are saying the same things in hushed tones at the same time. As NREM sleep becomes deeper, the whole stadium chants in union: *Go team go! Go team go!*

Dr. Kleitman discovered that the brain alternates between the relatively inactive NREM and highly active REM in a predictable fashion, with the brain cycling through both stages every 90 minutes or so. He also theorized that the 90-minute cycle is a fundamental unit of time for many of the body's other functions. He called this 90-minute cycle our basic rest and activity cycle, or the BRAC, a term mentioned earlier that remains in use today. The BRAC is a programmed inner clock that drives brain activity patterns and other physiological functions in a predictable and repetitive fashion over time. These clocks alternate periods of rest with periods of activity.

Over the decades, research has borne out Kleitman's theory. When people are placed in a room without the normal barrage of time cues from stimuli such as light, regularly timed meals, or television, they exhibit dozens of body functions running on a 90-minute cycle. For example, people engage in some kind of oral activity (eating, drinking, or smoking) every 90 minutes while waking. Patterns of electrical activity between the right and left hemispheres of the brain appear to alternate on a 90-minute cycle; various hormones, such as corticosterone, exhibit a stronger presence in the bloodstream every—you guessed it—90 minutes. Other body functions regulated by the 90-minute cycle include heart rate, urine flow, oxygen consumption, gastric motility (filling and emptying of the stomach), and nasal breathing patterns.

We also have 90-minute cycles of alertness during the day. Within this cycle, we have time for bright wakefulness, time for quiet focus, and time for daydreaming. When we adults come to the end of a 90-minute alertness cycle, we may experience a mild dip in attention—and then rev up again as we enter another 90-minute cycle.

For babies up to one year of age however, this 90-minute cycle is highly pronounced. At the end of each cycle, babies don't merely lose focus; they have built up what Alexander Borbély—director of the Sleep Laboratory of the Institute of Pharmacology at the University of Zurich—calls "sleep pressure" and need to discharge that pressure by going to sleep. Kleitman himself documented this pattern in his lab with his own eight-month-old baby. Many specialists, and I include myself, believe that if Kleitman had had access to today's powerful computer-based analysis programs, he could have isolated the pattern much earlier than eight months. Unfortunately, interest in lab research on babies' sleep has diminished in recent decades, and it's understandably difficult to persuade new parents to allow their babies to be monitored in a sleep laboratory. Yet the 90-minute cycle in infant rhythms, including phases of alertness, enjoys a widespread acceptability among sleep researchers, thanks to the remarkable consistency of the BRAC in so many other human functions. Human physiology is known for its variability and unpredictability—yet the BRAC *is* invariable, reassuringly always there, beating out its rhythm as reliably as a metronome. (The BRAC is also found in most other mammals with the same kind of consistency, although the length of the BRAC varies from species to species. Whereas humans run on 90-minute BRACs, a monkey's cycle is 72 minutes. A cat's is only 24 minutes!)

> **THE BRAC IS INVARIABLE, REASSURINGLY ALWAYS THERE, BEATING OUT ITS RHYTHM AS RELIABLY AS A METRONOME.**

I would like to see more studies on babies and the BRAC; however, I don't want to wait around for better funding to share what I've observed again and again in one-on-one experience with hundreds of parents and babies. This experience leads me to conclude that the 90-minute cycle is often present from birth—you can see a figure of a baby's 90-minute BRAC in the chart below—although there are some newborn babies who sleep on a shorter cycle until they grow into the full-length BRAC. By the time a

Baby's 90-Minute Basic Rest and Activity Cycle

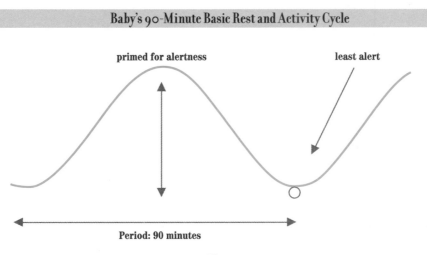

primed for alertness

least alert

Period: 90 minutes

baby reaches one year of age, sleep recordings begin to look more like those of an adult's, and in most cases the 90-minute cycle loses its grip on sleepy behavior. (In some children, the cycle appears to continue into toddlerhood.)

What does this mean for you? It means that *at the end of their alertness cycle, babies are ready to sleep.* This cycle is the basis of the N.A.P.S. plan.

"How Can the Baby Be Sleepy Again?"

I t bears repeating: *At the end of their alertness cycle, babies are ready to sleep.* The 90-minute timing is surprising and unsettling for many adults because a baby's window of alertness is so much shorter than our own. A mother may be astonished when her baby, who awoke at 7 o'clock in the morning, rubs his eyes and yawns at 8:30 AM. "How can the baby be sleepy?" she wonders. "He just slept all night!"

There's nothing wrong with the baby. In fact, he's right on target. As soon as a baby wakes up from sleep, his 90-minute clock starts running. Another fact that can surprise parents is that it doesn't matter how long the baby has slept prior to awakening. It's irrelevant whether he had a brief nap or a long night's slumber; either way, his 90-minute clock begins to tick as soon as he wakes up. And after 90 minutes of wakefulness, the baby has completed the alert phase governed by his inner clock. This is when the baby has the best chance of falling asleep quickly and easily. Again, the baby may be ready to take a nap or, if it's late in the day, to fall asleep for the night. Either way, if the parent is attuned to these phases and allows the baby to sleep when he is tired, the baby will be in harmony with his inner rhythm. This leads to sleep that is more restful and periods of alertness in which the baby is more focused.

Why Do Babies Need Help Following Their Cycles?

Parents are sometimes skeptical when they hear about the 90-minute cycle. "If it's so natural," they ask, "why don't babies simply close their eyes and go to sleep every 90 minutes?" It's an excellent question. One of the fascinating things about this body clock is that it doesn't actually induce sleep at a certain time. Instead, the clock governs wakefulness; it makes your baby *awake* at a certain time. Then, as the clock runs out, it withdraws alertness so sleep is possible.

This distinction is subtle, but it has important consequences for parents. We know it can be hard for adults, no matter how sleepy they are, to fall asleep in the middle of the morning or in the early evening when their own biological rhythms encourage them to be up and about. Babies can suffer from a similar problem. If you fail to help your baby fall asleep when the 90-minute alertness clock runs out, another cycle of alertness will start up again—and although your baby will be tired, the 90-minute clock will be busy promoting wakefulness. It will be very difficult for your baby to fall asleep until the cycle reaches its end and the next natural lull in alertness occurs. That's why it's so important for parents to keep track of the cycle (we'll cover this in greater detail later). If you overlook your baby's signs of fatigue or misinterpret them as a need for extra stimulation, you may miss the opportunity to help your little

IT'S SO IMPORTANT FOR PARENTS TO KEEP TRACK OF THE CYCLE. IF YOU OVERLOOK YOUR BABY'S SIGNS OF FATIGUE OR MISINTERPRET THEM AS A NEED FOR EXTRA STIMULATION, YOU MAY MISS THE OPPORTUNITY TO HELP YOUR LITTLE ONE SLEEP, AND YOU'LL END UP WITH A DRAMATICALLY OVERTIRED BABY.

one sleep, and you'll end up with a dramatically overtired baby.

Another reason babies don't simply drift off at the end of each cycle is related to one of the fundamental differences between a baby's sleep and our own. Falling asleep seems natural to adults, so natural that an inability to fall asleep is often considered a medical condition to be treated with behavioral therapy or drugs. Imagine if we fell asleep only while riding around in the backseat of a car—as so many babies do—or while someone rocked us back and forth!

But young babies (especially those in the first six months of life) are still in the midst of extensive neural development, and many of them are not yet ready to fall asleep on their own. There are some exceptions, of course. We've all heard stories about wonder babies who close their tiny eyelids at 7 PM and then sleep all the way through the night at two months of age. Those babies, however, are truly exceptions, and it's helpful to know that in the newborn months, the brain of a baby is not like the brain of an adult. As adults, our perceptions of the world are fully intact. We have lots of short-cut understandings about the world and the things in it. We know which sounds and sights and smells deserve our attention and which don't. Even in a crowded, noisy room, we can immediately pick out the sound of someone saying our name.

When we want to sleep, we can tune out the hum of the refrigerator, the weight of blankets on our skin, and the occasional digestive rumble.

Babies do not yet have this ability to tune out irrelevant or meaningless sensory information. Before they can learn what information is important and what to ignore, they must experience the world and everything in it, day by day. Engineers like to talk about something called a signal-to-noise ratio, which is the extent to which meaningful information can be understood against background noise. There's a lot of neural "noise" in a young baby's life. A baby has no choice but to take in all the sensations that bombard his brain and struggle to make sense of all this data. Amid all this information, it's hard for the baby to focus on the signal his brain is sending, telling him it's time to go to sleep.

In some ways, babies are like formerly blind adults who have surgically regained their sight. Newly sighted people are able to see colors and shapes and shadows—but they don't know what any of these things mean because they haven't had enough practice processing visual information and learning which bits of information they need to pay attention to. They don't understand which dark colors belong to an object and are part of it, for example, and which are shadows cast by the object. Life as a baby must be similarly confusing but on a much larger scale. Sights, textures, bodily sensations—even when he is tired and needs sleep, a baby is forced to pay attention to nearly every piece of information that comes his way.

We can only imagine how frustrating it must be for a baby who feels an urge to sleep but is helpless to act on it. That's one reason so many babies cry when they're sleepy. As adults, we shouldn't assume our crying babies are bored and in need of entertainment. Singing toys and brightly colored mobiles are exactly what they *don't* need at this time. Instead, it's up to us to provide a serene environment that includes repetitive motions, such as rocking back and forth, that allow babies to focus and calm down.

The 90-Minute Cycles in Your Baby's First Year

When it comes to patterns of sleep and wakefulness, the 90-minute clock is the basic unit of time in the brain for the first year of life. As your baby begins to initiate sleep in synchrony with this alertness clock, his sleep bouts will tend to last for multiples of 90 minutes. Although there is no hard-and-fast rule about nap length, you'll probably start to see naps that last either an hour and a half *or* three hours. Nighttime sleep will often occur in 90-minute multiples as well. In the newborn period, those multiples may be short, but as your baby grows older those nighttime sleep bouts will stretch into longer periods: four and a half hours, six hours, seven and a half hours, nine hours, ten and a half hours, or more.

As your baby continues to grow, the 90-minute clock is still in operation, but there will gradually be more and more periods in the day when he can stay awake for longer intervals: often for two consecutive 90-minute blocks of time (that is, three hours) or sometimes three consecutive 90-minute periods (four and a half hours). By the time your baby is one year old, the 90-minute clock generally has a less dramatic effect on sleep, although some parents will continue to see it in evidence. However, the 90-minute rhythm remains important throughout life.

Babies Who Follow Their 90-Minute Rhythms Develop Better Sleep Habits

When you learn to spot the 90-minute rhythm in your baby, you are on track to teaching him some important skills. He'll learn to identify his feelings of fatigue and know that sleep, not food or stimulation or crying, is the best response to those feelings. Because he'll wake up refreshed in the morning and after naps, he'll start to link that good feeling with having slept well. When a baby, even a newborn, falls asleep according to his biological rhythm, he is more likely to take satisfying naps and sleep for longer stretches at night. When his rapidly developing nervous system is ready, he'll reach the Holy Grail of infancy: sleeping all the way through until morning.

 WHEN A BABY, EVEN A NEWBORN, FALLS ASLEEP ACCORDING TO HIS BIOLOGICAL RHYTHM, HE IS MORE LIKELY TO TAKE SATISFYING NAPS AND SLEEP FOR LONGER STRETCHES AT NIGHT.

Eventually, when your baby is at an appropriate age (usually between six and eight months), the N.A.P.S. plan will help him learn how to fall asleep on his own. You may have heard grim stories about children who cry and protest for painfully long periods before learning sleep independence, but well-rested babies who follow their inner clocks tend to learn this skill quickly and easily, often with minimal or no crying. And although there's no denying that toddlers can be stubborn creatures, eager to assert their independence at bedtime, the N.A.P.S. plan decreases the chances of defiant bedtime wars, because babies who follow their rhythms are more likely to grow

Fern's Story: *A Very, Very Colicky Baby*

"**M**y daughter, Jessica, was a very, very colicky baby. She cried four or five hours during the day, sometimes longer. Nights were worse. Jessica would start crying at around five o'clock and keep crying until eleven or twelve. Then she'd go down for bed, but not for long. She'd wake up, I'd feed her and change her and get her back to sleep—and then she was up again half an hour later. I read seven books trying to understand what was wrong. Now I know she was sleep deprived.

"By the time Jessica was twelve weeks old, I was so tired I couldn't function. When I first heard about the 90-minute cycle, my first reaction was: There is no way this baby is going to sleep every 90 minutes. But I liked the idea of a gentle way to manage the baby's sleep and crying, so I decided to try it.

"Jessica had fallen asleep in the car on the way home from Polly's talk. When she woke up, I noted the time. About 90 minutes later, Jessica was crying, but she didn't look all that sleepy to me. I sat down with her in the rocking chair anyway, and we rocked back and forth as I held her. After about five minutes, Jessica was asleep and I put her down in her crib for a long nap. Needless to say, I kept using the N.A.P.S. plan. The other parents in Jessica's playgroup laughed at me for letting my daughter nap so often, but within a week, Jessica was sleeping through the night.

"Now Jessica is a toddler. Although she has outgrown the strict 90-minute cycle, I still pay close attention to her need for sleep—and she is one of the only babies in her playgroup who goes down for the night without a fuss. None of the other parents are giving me flak now. In fact, they come to me for advice about how to get their children to sleep."

into children who understand their own sleepiness. They may even *ask* to go to bed when they're tired!

Guide Your Child with Confidence

There are benefits for you as well. You'll get more sleep of your own, of course. You'll have more enjoyable time with your baby because a well-rested child is calmer, more focused, and cheerful. Perhaps best of all, the N.A.P.S. plan takes some of the guesswork out of parenting. All parents (and babysitters) know the frustration of trying to placate the mysterious wails of a child, first with toys, then with food, maybe with rides in the car—but if you keep an eye on the clock, you'll know when your baby is crying with fatigue. I'm always gratified when the parents I work with report greater confidence responding to their baby's needs.

The N.A.P.S. plan is easy to apply, as you'll see in the next chapter. In a few simple steps, you and your baby can start to enjoy the benefits of better sleep.

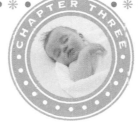
The N.A.P.S. Plan
The Basics

I created the N.A.P.S. plan to make following your baby's 90-minute cycles as straightforward as possible. The plan will help you remember what to do, when to do it, and how to spot the signals telling you that your baby is ready for sleep. The name of the plan is significant because your baby's internal clock is designed for frequent naps throughout the day. Babies whose parents are not sensitive to their napping needs tend to be crabby during the day, overaroused or hyperactive at night, and unable to sleep well at any time. This concept is difficult for some parents to appreciate—until they try the N.A.P.S. plan for themselves and discover that sleep during the day leads not just to a more content child: It leads to even more sleep at night.

HERE'S A QUICK BREAKDOWN OF THE N.A.P.S. PLAN:

N: Note the time of your baby's last waking.

A: Add 90 minutes.

P: Play and pursue other activities with your baby.

S: Soothe your baby to sleep.

As you can see, the N.A.P.S. plan has only four steps. None of these steps is hard to follow once you become attuned to the 90-minute cycles and your baby's signs that she is ready to sleep. By following the plan, you can provide the conditions for the perfect nap, one that takes place according to your baby's inner drive for sleep and lasts until the baby wakes up on her own.

Note the Time of Your Baby's Last Waking

The first step is to note the time of your baby's last waking. As soon as you hear your baby stirring, check the clock and record the time (the journal portion of this book, which begins on page 145, provides useful sleep logs for this purpose).

There's nothing particularly difficult about the first step of the N.A.P.S. plan, although it may require you to be a little more aware of clock time. This can feel odd to new parents, who—after the sleepless nights of late pregnancy, labor, delivery, and around-the-clock newborn duty—have been thrust into a world in which time has lost some of its old meaning. Nevertheless, make the effort to note the exact time.

Notice that this step does *not* ask you to wake your baby up from sleep at a predetermined time. This is in contrast to some popular advice, which people justify by saying that it allows a baby to sleep better at night or helps you maintain a predictable schedule. Of course, good nights and predictable days are important to the sanity of parents, but you won't achieve either by disturbing your baby's naps. Instead, let your baby awaken naturally. The N.A.F.S. plan works because it teaches your baby to follow her own internal rhythms, which include times for falling asleep and times for waking up.

SLEEP IS LIKE BREATHING. YOUR BABY CAN'T BREATHE TOO MUCH TODAY AND NOT NEED TO BREATHE TONIGHT. THE SAME GOES FOR SLEEP.

Waking naturally helps your baby's brain learn to do two things. One important job accomplished by sleep is to discharge the energy built up during wakefulness. A natural waking teaches the baby how to sleep until this and other neurological housekeeping tasks in the brain are completed. If the baby is frequently awakened artificially from her daytime naps, her brain doesn't get the same opportunity to learn these lessons, and the result is shorter sleep length—both at naps *and* at night. Even if you are concerned that a nap or morning sleep has gone on "too long," do not wake your sleeping baby. The same is true for toddlers, by the way—and it would be a wonderful world if teenagers and adults could also arise according to their own rhythms instead of alarm clocks. Think of it this way: Sleep is like breathing. Your baby can't breathe too much today and not need to breathe tonight. The same goes for sleep.

There are exceptions to the don't-wake-a-sleeping-baby rule. Low-birthweight babies and others with special needs may need to be awakened from sleep in order to eat. Your pediatrician will tell you if your baby's nutritional needs trump the benefits of waking naturally, and of course you should always follow his or her advice. Other circumstances, such as travel across time zones or the management of schedules for twins or triplets, may justify wakings. These situations are described more fully starting on page 173.

Of course, there will be times in everyday life with a healthy single-ton baby when you absolutely need to disturb a nap—to get to a doctor's appointment, perhaps, or to pick up an older sibling at school. There's not much you can do about these events, so don't feel guilty about them. We parents can be in only one place at a time. But don't wake up the baby just because Grandpa wants to play with her or because you're tired of waiting around for the nap to end. You, Grandpa, and the baby will all have a much more enjoyable time together when the baby is fully rested.

Add 90 Minutes

Take the time that you've just noted (the time of the baby's last waking) and add 90 minutes. Write this number down because it tells you when your baby will be ready to sleep again. For example, if your baby woke up from her nap at 10:00 AM, you can expect the next nap to occur at around 11:30 AM. The 90-minute rule holds true no mat-ter how long the baby's previous sleep period lasted. If she slept from 9:40 AM until 10:00 AM, she'll be ready for sleep again at 11:30. If she slept from 7:00 AM until 10:00 AM, she'll also be ready for sleep again at 11:30. Why? Because *at the end of their alertness cycle, babies are naturally ready to sleep.*

As I mentioned earlier in this book, your baby will extend some of her wakeful periods starting at around four months or so. These longer windows of alertness usually last for either three hours (or two consecutive 90-minute intervals) or four and a half hours (or three consecutive 90-minute intervals). You can read more about these changes on pages 82 to 84 and 94.

Play

Now that your baby is awake, it's a good time for a diaper change and a feeding. I suggest feeding your baby early in the 90-minute interval, instead of at the end of it when it will be harder to distinguish hunger fussing from sleepy fussing. Feeding your baby when she is wide awake also means she is more likely to eat heartily and to the point of satisfaction, instead of dozing off before her stomach is full. Babies who take a snack-and-nibble approach to feedings are much more likely to wake up at night, expecting food at frequent intervals.

Now that your baby has all her basic needs met, she's ready to play. If you're a first-time parent, it can be surprising to find that babies who are just a few weeks old don't play in a way that we recognize. They don't grab toys or giggle or even smile yet. But they do enjoy a short window of quiet alertness. You can hold them, sing or talk to them, or just let them take in the world. Older babies may enjoy a few rounds of the song "The Wheels on the Bus," investigating their surroundings, or manipulating simple toys.

This is also a good time to run errands. Your well-rested baby is open to the world and primed for gentle stimulation. Going on trips to the dry cleaner, the grocery store, or to visit friends gives your baby a glimpse of life outside the nursery. Just be aware that your baby cannot comfortably stay awake for very long. True, it's hard to run several errands within the space of 90 minutes, but the 90-minute clock is a biological fact, not a parental choice. All young babies are designed to get sleepy after 90 minutes, whether or not their parents understand their biological need for sleep. Running errands with a tired baby who fusses at the bank and then falls asleep in the car—and wakes up screaming when you park at the grocery store a few minutes later—is neither productive nor fun. It's much more pleasant for both of you to break up your activities into small segments that you and baby can manage. You'll be surprised at how often strangers will smile and say, "What a happy little baby you have!"

Anne's Story: *A Lucky Mother?*

"I've been following the N.A.P.S. plan since my daughter was born. When I visit my family, they say, 'You let your baby nap too much!' Then, in practically the next breath, they say, 'You're lucky to have such a good little baby!' I do have a happy baby, but luck has nothing to do with it. She's happy because I let her sleep before she gets too cranky. If we miss a nap, look out: She cries as much as all the other babies we know."

Soothe Your Sleepy Baby

A critical step in the N.A.P.S. plan is knowing when the 90-minute clock is running out, with your baby at the end of the alertness phase. This is when your baby has the best chance of falling asleep easily and staying asleep for a good long stretch. So it's in your and your baby's best interest to identify when the cycle is at its low point. Take another look at the illustration on page 28 and you'll see what I mean. This is when it's time to soothe your baby and prepare her for sleep.

The easiest way to keep track of the 90-minute cycle is to watch the clock. You've already noted the time of your baby's last waking and added 90 minutes. When you approach this time, get ready to soothe your baby in preparation for sleep. How do you know exactly when to start soothing your baby? In addition to watching the clock, also watch your baby for signs of sleepiness, which I'll describe in the next paragraph. Those signs of sleepiness will probably occur just a few minutes before the 90-minute cycle is over, and they tell you that the time is ripe to usher your baby into slumber. If you follow these cues, you may find your baby is asleep, or almost asleep, within moments after you begin your comforting ritual.

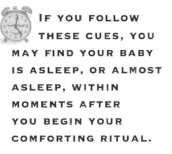 **IF YOU FOLLOW THESE CUES, YOU MAY FIND YOUR BABY IS ASLEEP, OR ALMOST ASLEEP, WITHIN MOMENTS AFTER YOU BEGIN YOUR COMFORTING RITUAL.**

Spotting the signs of sleepiness sounds easy, but it can be a little tricky. After all, it's not as if your baby can say, "I'm tired, Mom. Toss me my blankie and get me to my crib, pronto!" And if you expect sleepy babies to show the same signs of fatigue—yawning, rubbing their eyes, or looking droopy lidded—as adults do, you may miss your baby's cues altogether. That's because babies have their own special ways of exhibiting sleepy behavior, and these behaviors tend to be different from yours and mine. Some are physical, some are emotional, and some affect a baby's ability to focus and pay attention. Some babies do yawn or rub their eyes (if they have the motor skills), but many simply cry or look off into the middle distance. The chart below lists the most common sleepy signs. Your baby may show just one or several at once; she may also have additional sleepy signs that are not on this chart. (My daughter, Maddie, had an unusual sleepy sign I haven't seen in any other baby: She curled her hands into fists and drew her arms back. Her face also looked different, as if it were drained of emotion.) I encourage you to note your baby's own signals in the journal section of this book, pages 145 to 172.

You may notice your baby's sleepy signs a bit early, perhaps as early as 70 minutes or so into the cycle. In this case, it's probably not the cycle that's off. It's just that your baby woke up and started running the clock earlier than you realized. Some babies wake quietly and play or take in their surroundings for a while before making a peep. That's why you

Common Sleepy Signals				
PHYSICAL	Rubbing eyes, either with hands or on the carpet or against someone's shoulder	Pulling on ears	Yawning	
EMOTIONAL	Crying	Whining (especially when not being held)	Cranked-up, hyper behavior	Suddenly becoming frustrated or impatient
ATTENTIONAL	Appearing spacey, unresponsive, or withdrawn	Suddenly losing interest in a toy or activity		

need to become attuned to your baby's signals in addition to watching the clock. As soon as you note the sleepy signs ("There's my signal!"), begin to soothe your baby. If your baby isn't giving off any sleep signals

> **IF YOUR BABY ISN'T GIVING OFF ANY SLEEP SIGNALS YOU CAN RECOGNIZE, START SOOTHING FIVE OR TEN MINUTES BEFORE THE 90-MINUTE CYCLE IS OVER.**

you can recognize, start soothing five or ten minutes before the 90-minute cycle is over.

If you currently soothe your baby until she is sound asleep, continue to do so for now. (Remember that most babies who are younger than six months old need an adult's help to fall asleep.) If you have an older baby who already knows how to fall asleep on her own, you can begin the soothing process and then put her down while she's drowsy but still awake.

If your baby is just a few days or weeks old, or if she is sick, you may notice she wants to sleep more frequently than every 90 minutes. That's fine. *Don't try to keep your baby awake when she's sending out sleepy signals.* (Sometimes babies become very sleepy when they are sick or injured. You know your baby best; if she seems unusually sleepy to you, call your doctor.)

What's the best way to soothe sleepy babies? By making their environment comfortingly monotonous, so some of the sensory "noise" from the outside world is drowned out. This usually means performing a rocking or other repetitive motion: sitting in a rocking chair with the baby or walking with the baby in your arms or in a sling. Babies who have spent nine months or so being rocked in the womb by your movements understand this rhythm and repetition. Your warmth, as well as your familiar voice and scent, will also help comfort your baby. You may find that your baby cries just when you begin rocking and soothing, but don't give up immediately. Stick with it, gently. Your baby may soon quiet down and enjoy the motion.

Be wary of exhausting techniques—you want the baby to be sleepy, but you don't want to tire yourself out! Parents sometimes

SOOTHING TECHNIQUES

Recommended soothing techniques *(to be used as often as you like):*

- Rocking the baby back and forth

- Swinging the baby back and forth in your arms (make sure you maintain complete control of your movements)

- Walking with the baby in your arms or in a sling

- Swaying gently back and forth while holding the baby

- Swaddling the baby in a light receiving blanket (you'll probably need to use motion in addition to swaddling)

- Singing or making a hushing sound (hearing the same song or sound over and over gives the baby something to focus on)

Soothing techniques that are not recommended for regular use *(save these for special circumstances):*

- Driving the baby around in the car

- Walking the baby in a stroller

- Placing the baby in a swing

- Feeding (use this only in the newborn period as a sleep inducer; if your baby is three months or older, try to use other methods as often as you can) stumble onto methods such as dancing with their babies or doing deep knee bends while holding the child in their arms—but as you might imagine, these strategies quickly lose their charm (for the parents, anyway) even as the baby grows to depend on them for sleep. A sooth-

BE WARY OF EXHAUSTING TECHNIQUES—YOU WANT THE BABY TO BE SLEEPY, BUT YOU DON'T WANT TO TIRE YOURSELF OUT!

ing technique that wears you out probably isn't going to work for very long. On the other end of the spectrum are techniques like taking the baby for a ride in the car or stroller, or placing the baby in a swing. Your baby may be easily consoled by these mechanical devices, but she can get addicted to them and be unable to fall asleep any other way. You don't want to have to drive around the block or haul out the swing every time the baby awakes at night. Reserve these strategies for when you really need them, such as when the baby is sick or nothing else is working, and try not to depend on them.

Nursing or giving the baby a bottle can have a calming, center-ing effect on a tired baby. But don't *always* rely on feeding your baby to sleep. In the early weeks it may be difficult to determine whether your baby is hungry or sleepy, and that's okay, but eventually—around three months of age—you'll want your baby to understand that the appropriate response to sleepiness is sleep, not food. One advantage of the N.A.P.S. plan is that your baby will drift off to sleep more easily—without depending on nursing, stroller rides, or swings—when you time her sleep properly.

Mystery Fussiness

Avery tired baby will probably be wound up and agitated, perhaps crying hard. If you have ever felt so tired that you couldn't fall asleep, you know what an unpleasant state this is. All a tired baby knows is that she feels terrible, and she needs you to help her.

Sometimes in my classes I refer to this state as "mystery fussiness." I present the following scenario to parents and ask if it has ever happened to them: *Your baby is fussing, and you can't figure out why. You've tried everything you can think of—feeding, changing the diaper, giving her a new toy—but the fussiness never stops for long. Then, when you're completely boggled, you feed the baby once more, not because you think she's hungry, but because you've simply run out of options. Within seconds of starting to feed the baby, you notice with relief that your baby has fallen fast asleep.*

THIS IS A "LIGHT BULB" MOMENT FOR MANY IN THE AUDIENCE WHEN THEY REALIZE MYSTERY FUSSINESS IS OFTEN A SIGN OF SLEEPINESS IN BABIES.

As I describe the situation, hands go up from virtually every parent in the room, with vigorous nodding from some. Then I ask: Was the baby crying because she was hungry or because she was sleepy? This is a "light bulb" moment for many in the audience when they realize mystery fussiness is often a sign of sleepiness in babies. Maybe this is a light bulb moment for you too. Babies cry not just when they are hungry or wet or bored. They also cry because they're tired.

They *often* cry because they're tired. Yet ofter this piece of information is omitted from new-parent education. A veteran pediatrician once told me that babies cry for one of ten reasons: hunger, loneliness, gas, a wet diaper, a soiled diaper, discomfort, boredom, sickness, teething pain, or other pain. I was shocked that fatigue didn't make the list. One mother I know was struggling with her newborn because the child's grandmother insisted that crying meant the baby must be cold, sick, or not getting enough milk. The mother found herself feeding the baby whenever she cried—which was every 90 minutes. She had recognized the cycle but hadn't realized that crying could be a sign of sleepiness.

So why does feeding help tired babies sleep? The act of feeding and sucking is very focusing for babies and helps them calm down—and it's why so many of us parents understandably become dependent on feeding to get our babies to sleep. Of course, it's not wrong to feed your baby! But when you recognize the signs of sleepiness in your child, you can then respond with the most appropriate action—helping her sleep—instead of frantically running through the feed-change-play gamut first, as the child grows more and more distressed.

There are other light bulb moments, such as when a baby who seems to "hate" the supermarket and cries at the checkout counter suddenly falls asleep in the car seat on the trip home. It's a great relief to realize the fussiness isn't caused by the excursion itself but by fatigue. Now you know what to do: Avoid running errands when the baby is sleepy. Wait until nap time is over.

Enjoy the N.A.P.S.

Now you can enjoy your baby's nap time. Get some sleep yourself, if you can. Don't underestimate how hard you are working both day and night. Parenthood can sometimes feel like an extended experiment in sleep deprivation. If you can't rest (your own alertness rhythms may prevent you from napping during the day), take advantage of the baby's

NOW YOU CAN ENJOY YOUR BABY'S NAP TIME. GET SOME SLEEP YOURSELF.

sleep time to do the things you can't do while your baby is awake. Read a book, exercise, attempt a project that requires unbroken concentration, or do chores that involve heavy lifting or going up and down the stairs repeatedly. Remember to allow your baby to awaken naturally. Then start the 90-minute clock, and the N.A.P.S. plan, all over again.

N.A.P.S. at Night

Just as babies experience 90-minute cycles of alertness, it takes roughly 90 minutes for most babies to go through all the stages of sleep, depending on their age and level of development. In this way, they are developing some of the sleep characteristics of adults, who also take 90 minutes to cycle through the stages of sleep. At the end of each 90-minute sleep cycle, the brain undergoes a kind of system check in which it is partially aroused. Sleep scientists believe we all experience little pseudo-awakenings at night, especially during these system checks. We adults rarely recall these awakenings later because we usually resume sleeping without incident or interruption. Babies seem to have these mini-wakings as well. When they are well rested from getting proper naps during the day, babies may crack an eye open, maybe roll over if they're able . . . and then, with a little luck, peacefully return to sleep.

But not all babies are able to get back to sleep so easily. In fact, the 90-minute sleep cycle helps explain why some babies wake up crying at night. Sometimes babies cry because they are hungry, but they may also cry because their nervous systems are still immature. Their neurological "system check" can register an imbalance and wake them up. Things are worse for babies who don't get proper naps. These babies build up extra energy that should have been discharged during day sleep, making their nervous systems even more likely to tilt toward irritability and imbalance. That's why nap-deprived babies have so many partial night awakenings that turn into full-blown wake-ups. This waking is often accompanied by crying because they want someone to help them return to the sleep state they crave.

BY FOLLOWING THE N.A.P.S. PLAN AND GIVING YOUR BABY SUFFICIENT SLEEP IN THE DAY, YOU GIVE HER THE BEST CHANCE AT DRIFTING BACK TO SLEEP ON HER OWN AT NIGHT.

With a very young baby, it's appropriate to feed, comfort, or soothe a crying child back to sleep at night. But even during this early period, there are steps you can take to encourage good night sleep. By following the N.A.P.S. plan and giving your baby sufficient sleep in the day, you give her the best chance at drifting back to sleep on her own at night. Older babies are even more likely to show the nighttime benefits of plentiful daytime sleep.

Frequently Asked Questions About the N.A.P.S. Plan

B ecause it is based on biological timekeeping, the N.A.P.S. plan works. Nevertheless, it goes so far against popular misconceptions about infant sleep that it's only natural to feel some skepticism. Here are the questions people ask most frequently about the plan.

DO I HAVE TO STAY HOME FOR THE BABY'S NAPS?

✳ The hardest part of the N.A.P.S. plan is that it requires a commitment to your baby's need for frequent naps. Earlier I described the "perfect nap," which is a nap that starts when your baby is tired and ends when she is done sleeping. How you achieve this napping perfection, and to what extent you'll have to restrict your activities, depends on your baby and where she sleeps best. Newborn babies are pretty good at sleeping almost anywhere, but many older babies don't seem to get a good rest unless they are in their own special sleeping quarters, usually a crib. If that's the case with your baby, you'll want to be home for naps. I understand that this may sound a little daunting to new parents who are used to coming and going as they please; it may make you feel better to ask your own parents what they did while you were napping. Chances are, they stayed home and let you sleep.

You may be able to create some flexibility. If you have a baby who is capable of sleeping in environments other than her crib (some babies are more adaptable than others), you might as well take advantage of this talent. I know a couple whose baby sleeps well in her car seat and does not wake up when the car stops, as many babies do. Their child takes most of her naps in her crib, but once a day they run errands, timing them so the baby falls asleep on the way home. They leave their daughter in her car seat in the front hallway with the baby monitor on, instead of jostling her upstairs to her crib. The baby wakes up when she is ready, and everyone is happy. Other parents keep portable playpens, Moses baskets, or portable cribs in the car, so the baby can sleep in a quiet room while the parents visit with friends.

No matter what, you will have to make changes to your routine and the way you plan your activities. Some parents find this frustrating at first, especially if they are eager to resume a social life after bed rest during pregnancy or if they experience pressure to take the baby out to meet with friends or family. But most people who try the N.A.P.S. plan conclude that life with N.A.P.S. is easier than life without it. Even though N.A.P.S. parents put their babies down to rest more frequently, they spend less total time each day on the comforting/soothing process, which can stretch into hours with a chronically fatigued baby. Everyone in the family is in a brighter mood and more able to take advantage of the baby's alert time to get out and enjoy life outside the home. Besides, the program lets parents get what they most desperately desire, which is a chance to put their feet up and rest. After all, they need to store up energy for the toddler years! Convenience aside, the N.A.P.S. plan allows your baby to meet one of her basic biological

> **CONVENIENCE ASIDE, THE N.A.P.S. PLAN ALLOWS YOUR BABY TO MEET ONE OF HER BASIC BIOLOGICAL NEEDS: SLEEP. ONCE YOU'VE SEEN YOUR BABY THRIVE ON THE N.A.P.S. PLAN, YOU'D NO MORE DEPRIVE HER OF A NAP THAN LET HER SKIP A FEEDING.**

NAPPING AWAY FROM HOME

When life interferes with your plan to let the baby take a nap at home, there are some ways to give your baby sleep anyway:

- If your errands or visits take you to a place where there's a quiet room, bring along a portable place to sleep. A playpen, Moses basket, or a portable crib can all work well. Try keeping one of these items in your car so you always have one on hand.

- If you often visit the baby's grandparents or other relatives, consider asking them to invest in an inexpensive (but sturdy and safe) crib or playpen that your baby can use for naps. Or buy one for them.

- Time your errands so the baby can fall asleep in the car on the way home. This works only if your baby sleeps well in the car and doesn't wake up when the car stops.

- Schedule your time so you can take the baby out in the stroller for a nap. Again, this works if you can keep walking, or at least stay within close reach of the stroller, until the baby finishes sleeping.

- Depending on where your outings take you, try wearing your baby in a front pack or sling for a nap.

- If you're in a place where you can sit quietly for a while, let your baby nap in your arms. This may be the easiest and most practical solution of all; plus, it gives you some time to doze off.

needs: sleep. Once you've seen your baby thrive on the N.A.P.S. plan, you'd no more deprive her of a nap than let her skip a feeding.

WILL MY BABY TAKE SHORTER NAPS ON THIS PROGRAM?

* Frequent naps do not make a baby's sleep periods shorter. Usually the opposite holds true: Babies who fall asleep according to their internal rhythms are less likely to suffer from premature awakenings during naps as well as at night. And because babies on the N.A.P.S. plan tend to stop falling asleep unexpectedly in the car seat, they are less prone to developing the catnaps that are often associated with car-seat sleeping.

WILL MY BABY SLEEP LESS AT NIGHT?

* The N.A.P.S. plan will actually help your baby sleep longer at night. Babies who don't get all their naps will tend to wake up irritable at night—usually after 90 minutes or a multiple of 90 minutes, such as three hours.

DO ALL BABIES REALLY FOLLOW THE 90-MINUTE CYCLE?

* As parents, we're often told that no single rule is true for all children. But remember that sleep, like food, is a basic need. If you think your baby doesn't need as much sleep as I suggest, give the plan a try anyway and see what happens. Babies who appear to need less sleep than other children are often truly underslept. Because they've suffered from chronic sleep loss, these babies generally need extra help drifting off to slumber or engaging in activities while awake.

However, there are some fluctuations in the 90-minute cycle across the first year of life. Many parents who are educated in the N.A.P.S. plan are able to see the 90-minute cycle even in their newborns. But it's also true that some newborn babies are unable to stay awake longer than

 BABIES WHO APPEAR TO NEED LESS SLEEP THAN OTHER CHILDREN ARE OFTEN TRULY UNDERSLEPT.

it takes to change and feed them; these children usually develop a 90-minute cycle sometime within the first weeks of life. Older babies

may double or triple the wakefulness cycle, so for a few times each day they are awake for periods that last 180 or 270 minutes (I'll describe these changes in the next two chapters). But no baby can escape the 90-minute sleep cycle completely.

WHAT IF I MISS THE 90-MINUTE WINDOW?

✳ If you miss the optimum chance for sleep at the end of the 90-minute phase, you may notice that your baby stops sending out sleepy signals. That's because the window of opportunity for sleep at the end of the 90-minute cycle is short. If the baby is not permitted to sleep, the 90-minute alertness clock starts up again, and your baby's brain revs up for another wakeful period, no matter how tired she is. Brace yourself, because you may now have a hyperaroused child on your hands. You will both pay the price—perhaps now, if the baby is wired and cranky, or later, if the baby misses so much daytime sleep that she's unable to rest well at night.

That's why it's so important to understand a baby's sleepy signals. When parents are not aware of sleepy signals, they may not respond to those signals appropriately. Instead, they are befuddled by what appears to be arbitrary fussiness. Then, as the window of opportunity closes, the sleepy signals end, and in most cases the baby will be unable to sleep until the next alertness cycle is completed.

When you find the 90-minute window has passed, you can try some soothing techniques anyway (see page 46). Perhaps your baby will be able to settle down and sleep for a while. If that doesn't work, keep an eye on the clock and get the soothing process underway at the end of the next 90-minute period.

If the baby is older, it's also possible that he is giving up one of his naps and making the transition to a 180- or 270-minute alertness cycle for part of the day.

WHAT IF I NEED TO LET MY BABY SKIP A NAP?

✳ To the extent possible, I recommend that you guard your baby's naps. Although of course you have many demands on your time, and deserve to have a life, establishing sound sleep habits is crucial to your baby's well-being. It's not fair to deprive your baby of sleep just because you don't like being tied to a schedule. But not even the most dedicated parent can be home for every single nap on every single day. There are school obligations, holiday dinners, family events, weddings, and other responsibilities that will interfere with the baby's schedule. In these circumstances, the N.A.P.S. plan still comes in handy. You'll be less surprised and more prepared for the exact times your baby will

> **ALTHOUGH OF COURSE YOU HAVE MANY DEMANDS ON YOUR TIME, AND DESERVE TO HAVE A LIFE, ESTABLISHING SOUND SLEEP HABITS IS CRUCIAL TO YOUR BABY'S WELL-BEING.**

become tired and require more holding and attention. With some luck, you may be able to duck out of a special event at the right time and keep her from fussing too loudly and disrupting a meal or a ceremony. Try to give your baby a nap whenever you get the chance . . . but keep in mind that when the 90-minute window of opportunity passes, the baby may start up another 90-minute cycle of alertness. You may have to wait until the end of *that* cycle before the baby will sleep again.

CAN CO-SLEEPING PARENTS USE THE N.A.P.S. PLAN?

✳ Co-sleeping is a practice in which babies are allowed to sleep in their parents' beds at night and often are worn in slings most of the day. Some parents co-sleep because small living quarters leave them no other choice, but many parents co-sleep for philosophical reasons. These parents feel that babies are more secure when they are physically close to their parents. They also feel strongly that it's unnatural to force babies onto a preprogrammed sleep schedule.

Co-sleeping is undeniably warm and delightful. It can also place heavy demands on parents. If you co-sleep, you may know the frustration of waiting—sometimes for hours—for your baby to "spontaneously" fall asleep. The N.A.P.S. plan can assist you by helping you identify the times when your baby is naturally ready to sleep and teaching you how to soothe (not force!) your baby into slumber. As a parent who maintains lots of close contact with your baby, you will probably find the plan very easy to follow because you have plenty of opportunity to observe your baby and learn her sleepy signals. Unlike other parents, however, you will probably not choose to put your baby down alone in a crib or bassinet to sleep. That's fine, as long as you are willing to nap with your baby or "wear" her in a sling until she's done sleeping.

A note about co-sleeping: There are some concerns about the safety of the practice. If you choose to co-sleep, I recommend you visit the American Academy of Pediatrics website, www.aap.org, or www.firstcandle.org for important sleep safety information.

DO FIXED SCHEDULES PROVIDE MORE SECURITY?

✳ Parents are often advised to put their babies on a schedule directed solely by clock time. This usually involves one nap at 9:00 AM and another at 1:00 PM, sometimes with a short third nap at around 4 or 5 o'clock in the evening for younger babies. Advocates of these schedules say that regular nap times help infants feel more secure. Another supposed advantage of clock schedules is that they teach babies the important lesson that parents are in charge of the family, and the baby must follow the parents' rules. Is there any truth to these claims?

Yes and no. Schedules are important for babies and their families, but the baby's inner clock needs to dictate the schedule. The amazing thing is that a baby's clock usually produces a predictable schedule by the age of six months or so if left to develop on its own. This biologically driven regularity is good for babies, but not just because it makes them feel secure. It's good for the babies because their sleep times match their inner clocks and the rhythms within their brains.

As for the claim that parents need to teach their babies who's in charge: It's important for parents to take a leadership role in the family, but they should do it in a way that matches the child's age and ability.

Ignoring a baby's need for sleep doesn't make the baby feel more secure; instead, an important element of security comes when a baby can trust that her parents will show her how to get sleep when she needs it. By following the N.A.P.S. plan, you'll have a baby who will grow into a well-rested child—the kind of child who is less likely to fight you over bedtimes and family rules and more likely to bloom into her happiest, best self.

Susan's Story: *A Noisy Sleepy Signal*

"My first child, Vincent, was born screaming, and it felt like he didn't stop for eight weeks. By the time Vincent was two months old, his crying had calmed somewhat, but he still seemed irritated a lot and didn't sleep nearly as much as the pediatrician said he should. At this point, I tried the N.A.P.S. plan. I knew I was supposed to look for Vincent's sleepy signs after 90 minutes of alertness, but at first I couldn't see them. It took a few days before I realized that Vincent showed his sleepy sign (crying) much earlier than other children: He would start to fuss 60 or 70 minutes into the cycle. I would hold him and rock him, but he wouldn't close his eyes until exactly 90 minutes after waking. It was uncanny. Vincent was so sensitive that he needed more time to wind down than other babies.

"As the months passed, Vincent spent less time crying. When he was about six months old, he'd start fussing at around 80 minutes into the cycle and then fall asleep at the 90-minute mark. People thought I was nuts for being so precise about his fussing and sleep times—but I was beyond caring. Vincent followed a timetable that was clear to me, my husband, and anyone else who tracked his behavior."

CHAPTER FOUR

The N.A.P.S. Plan
Birth Through Five Months

A cross the first year of life. the N.A.P.S. plan remains basically the same. Within this year, however, there are several developmental stages, and predictable changes and challenges occur at each one. In this chapter, you'll learn how to use the N.A.P.S. plan in a way that's age appropriate for your baby from birth through his first half-year of life, marked by his six-month birthday.

Many new parents wonder how often and how much their baby should sleep during naps and at night and how those amounts change as the baby grows. In Chapter 1 there is a sleep-distribution chart that tracks average sleep amounts across the first two years. Remember that this chart describes the *average* baby not *all* babies. Don't worry about trying to make your baby conform precisely to these charts. It's much more important to let your baby's sleep signals be your guide and to make sure he is allowed to sleep whenever he is tired. Focus on reading your baby, not the sleep charts. It's a far more pleasant and effective approach to good sleep.

Birth to Two Weeks

Babies sleep a *lot* in the first two weeks. To an adult, a new baby's sleep amounts can seem almost absurd: sixteen, eighteen, twenty, or even more hours each day. When babies are in the womb, they sleep most of the time, and the first two weeks of life are an extension of that very sleepy stage.

In the first two weeks, you may find that the baby will sometimes fall asleep without much intervention from you. Babies at this stage can conk out practically anywhere—in the bassinet, in the car seat, in your arms, or even on the floor of a playpen. They also sleep like rocks. Newborns can sleep through the sounds of garbage disposals, loud music, and ambulance sirens. With some temperamentally easy babies who sleep a great deal and for several hours at a time, parenthood can seem like a piece of cake in those first few weeks. Do not be lulled into a false sense of complacency! Get all the rest you can while you can, because soon your baby's waking mechanisms will kick in.

WHEN BABIES ARE IN THE WOMB, THEY SLEEP MOST OF THE TIME, AND THE FIRST TWO WEEKS OF LIFE ARE AN EXTENSION OF THAT VERY SLEEPY STAGE.

WHAT'S SO HARD ABOUT A BABY WHO SLEEPS ALL THE TIME?

✳ Of course, not everyone finds these first couple of weeks so easy. It's normal to feel great physical and emotional stress as moms (and dads) recover from the demands of pregnancy and childbirth and adjust to their new role as parent. And although breastfeeding offers great rewards for you and your baby, and yields some of life's most tender moments, many mothers who are new to breastfeeding often find it hard work at first.

Even babies who sleep twenty hours a day can be a challenge to care for. It's not as if they sleep for twenty hours straight! Instead, they nod off for periods that usually last somewhere from twenty minutes to four hours, or possibly more. You, the parent, also have to snatch your sleep in bits and pieces.

As you observe your baby in these early weeks, remember that babies need to be fed frequently—but also remember that babies can wake up for reasons other than hunger. They may wake up simply because one of their sleep cycles has ended and they cannot transition back to sleep without help from an adult. Later, you can use this knowledge to condition your baby to sleep longer. For now, though, feed your baby whenever he appears to demand it.

LOOK FOR THE 90-MINUTE CYCLE

✳ Start looking for the 90-minute cycle now, but don't be discouraged if it doesn't emerge right away. It's not clear whether all babies exhibit the 90-minute cycle during these earliest weeks of life. Some babies are born with a 90-minute alertness clock clearly in place. I could spot a

90-minute alertness period in my second child, Max, while he was still in the hospital. About 90 minutes after awaking, he'd start to cry, and I knew to help him sleep. Other babies have shorter periods of wakefulness, and that's fine too.

Here's what I recommend for parents of newborns: First of all, don't force your baby to stay awake for 90 minutes if he is sleepy earlier. (This is true for your baby's entire first year, not just the first two weeks.) I also recommend against pushing your new baby onto any rigid feeding or sleeping schedule, unless there's a medical reason for doing so. I do recommend you try to pay attention to the time of his awakenings if you can, although I know in these early weeks it's not easy. This way, if your new baby starts to cry an hour or an hour and a half after his last waking, you'll have a good idea what the fuss is about: He's sleepy. You can then use your preferred soothing techniques to help him sleep.

START LOOKING FOR THE 90-MINUTE CYCLE NOW, BUT DON'T BE DISCOURAGED IF IT DOESN'T EMERGE RIGHT AWAY. IT'S NOT CLEAR WHETHER ALL BABIES EXHIBIT THE 90-MINUTE CYCLE DURING THESE EARLIEST WEEKS OF LIFE.

If you're able to track the baby's wake-up times and spot the alertness cycle, you'll avoid the horror stories so often told about newborn babies: "My baby cries nonstop," or "My baby cried for three straight hours last night." When I hear these statements, I think to myself, "That poor tired baby!" These experiences, miserable for both baby and parents, are unnecessary and, fortunately, avoidable. At least half of those three hours of crying could have been avoided if the parents had known to start soothing their baby after 90 minutes of wakefulness.

Even if you don't see a clear rhythm, it helps to know that babies cry from fatigue, just as they cry from hunger or discomfort. If your baby is fed, warm, and dry but is crying, don't try to distract him with toys or stimulation. Try helping your baby sleep instead. And don't be too hard on yourself. It's normal to be confused sometimes about whether your brand-new baby is hungry or sleepy or cold or wet. Do your best, and soon enough, your baby's cues will become clearer. The main things to remember are that babies at this age need to sleep a great deal, and when they are sleepy, they will probably cry for you to help them.

> **IF YOUR BABY IS FED, WARM, AND DRY BUT IS CRYING, DON'T TRY TO DISTRACT HIM WITH TOYS OR STIMULATION. TRY HELPING YOUR BABY SLEEP INSTEAD.**

DAY/NIGHT CONFUSION

✳ Newborns sometimes have their days and nights mixed up, with their longest sleep periods occurring during the daylight hours. This is normal and usually corrects itself in a few weeks as the baby's circadian rhythms emerge. (If that doesn't happen, see pages 133 to 134 for how gently to adjust the baby's rhythm to match yours a little more closely.) Waking your baby up from these long daytime naps will not, in all likelihood, encourage better sleep at night. This is important for a variety of reasons, some of which I've explained earlier. By letting your baby sleep for as long as he wants, even during the day, you are giving him the chance to learn how to extend and consolidate sleep on his own. You'll appreciate this ability to extend sleep in a few weeks when day/night confusion ends and those longer sleep periods start to appear at night.

BY LETTING YOUR BABY SLEEP FOR AS LONG AS HE WANTS, EVEN DURING THE DAY, YOU ARE GIVING HIM THE CHANCE TO LEARN HOW TO EXTEND AND CONSOLIDATE SLEEP ON HIS OWN.

When your baby does wake up at night, make sure you behave in a way that signals "nighttime." Use minimal lighting and speak in a hushed tone, even if you are wide awake. Parents who try to get through these middle-of-the-night awakenings by turning on all the lights, turning up the television, and speaking in daytime voices do not give the baby any reason to think that night is different from any other time. Thus they inadvertently give social cues that confuse the baby's developing circadian clock. In a similar fashion but in the reverse direction, parents who keep the house dark and silent all day may be hindering the development of appropriate day/ night patterns.

One way to manage nighttime tasks without lighting up the whole room is to use a red-bulb night light. This light will help you see well enough to safely feed and diaper the baby, but the long wavelengths of light (which we see as the color red) appear not to reset the circadian clock in the way that white bulbs do, and they are less stimulating to your baby's alertness mechanisms. You may need to take out the white bulb that comes with most night lights and replace it with a small red bulb that you've bought at a hardware store or a discount retailer.

ACTIVE SLEEP: DON'T LET IT TRICK YOU

✳ Newborn babies spend a much higher percentage of their sleep in the REM stage than we adults do. This highly active stage of sleep can look a lot like wakefulness or disturbed sleep to the adult observer. If your sleeping baby twitches, makes faces, or moves his eyes under half-open eyelids, don't worry—and try not to rush to pick him up. This behavior looks odd, but it is normal during REM sleep, and your baby is not suffering or having nightmares. Give the baby a chance to remain asleep and cycle on to the next sleep stage.

Young babies also spend a lot of time in a hazy in-between sleep stage that infant sleep specialists somewhat whimsically call "indeterminate." Like REM, the indeterminate stage can seem a lot like true wakefulness, but it may not be. In this stage, your baby may make some vocalizations, as if he is trying to talk to you. His eyelids may be closed but flickering, or you may see his eyes darting rapidly about under half-closed lids, or he may even have his eyes open.

YOUNG BABIES ALSO SPEND A LOT OF TIME IN A HAZY IN-BETWEEN SLEEP STAGE THAT INFANT SLEEP SPECIALISTS SOMEWHAT WHIMSICALLY CALL "INDETERMINATE." LIKE REM, THE INDETERMINATE STAGE CAN SEEM A LOT LIKE TRUE WAKEFULNESS, BUT IT MAY NOT BE.

Your impulse may be to greet the baby and pick him up, but be careful. He may not be fully awake and in fact may be able to transition back into "real" sleep, if you let him. You can try standing behind the baby, avoiding direct eye contact (because eye contact will surely wake him up if he isn't awake already), and give your baby a few minutes to try to return to sleep. If your baby is not fully awake and is able to drift back into a deeper sleep, he may eventually learn how to stretch his sleep into longer bouts.

THE N.A.P.S. PLAN AT A GLANCE

Birth to Two Weeks

- Expect your baby to sleep between fourteen and twenty hours per day. Sixteen hours is considered average; of course, all babies won't sleep this exact amount. Some will sleep more, and some will sleep less. It may even vary somewhat from day to day. This sleep will be scattered in short bursts across the day and night.

- Your baby will have very short periods of comfortable alertness. These may last for 90 minutes, or they may be shorter (sometimes the 90-minute cycle doesn't emerge until the baby gets a bit older). Don't encourage your baby to stay awake when he seems sleepy.

- Most babies at this age have not yet developed their individual sleepy signals. If they have not appeared yet, they will develop over the next few months. In these early weeks especially, your baby will probably cry when he is tired.

- Sometimes your newborn may be able to fall asleep on his own, without any assistance, but it's too early to expect your baby to always fall asleep independently. If he needs your help to sleep, use whatever soothing strategy works best for your baby. Recommendations for soothing can be found on pages 45 to 47.

- If your sleeping baby makes faces, thrashes about, "talks," or even opens his eyes without crying, don't rush to pick him up. He may be in an active stage of sleep; even if he's semi-awake, he may be able to pass back into sleep on his own.

- Take advantage of this relatively quiet period (and try not to brag about it!) because your baby will soon require more attention and soothing.

Two Weeks to Three Months

B y two weeks of age, babies still sleep quite a bit: around fifteen or sixteen hours daily and sometimes more. Nevertheless, this period is one of the most difficult times in parenting. That's because after the first few weeks, babies emerge from nearly constant sleep and start to show great displeasure at being awake. Babies who could once fall asleep on the living room carpet may now seem touchy and inflexible. As luck would have it, this very fussy time usually happens just as your spouse is heading back to work and any family members who've come by to help you get through the first few weeks are packing up to go home. You can take some consolation in knowing that your baby's unhappiness isn't caused by anything you've done or not done.

EVEN WHEN THINGS SEEM VERY HARD, YOU CAN HOLD ON TO THE KNOWLEDGE THAT AFTER 90 MINUTES OF WAKEFUL TIME, YOUR BABY WILL BE PRIMED FOR SLEEP.

The good news is that as the crying kicks in, so does the 90-minute cycle. The predictability of this cycle will pull you through these rough weeks. When my second baby was in this stage, the 90-minute cycle was my lifeline to sanity. Even when things seem very hard, you can hold on to the knowledge that after 90 minutes of wakeful time, your baby will be primed for sleep. Follow the N.A.P.S. plan to help your baby shut out the stimulating world, wind down, and get the sleep he needs.

Start watching your baby for unique sleepy signals that may be developing. Most babies at this age continue to cry when they are tired; others yawn, look wilted, or take on a thousand-yard stare. Babies who are temperamentally easy may not give out strong sleep signals but will gratefully close their eyes and snooze if you give them the chance.

Your baby is still very young. For now it's perfectly acceptable to use feeding, car rides, swings, or other external sources for soothing your baby. But as your baby reaches the end of the two- to three-month period, you'll want to reduce your reliance on these techniques and use others (such as rocking in a rocking chair, one of my favored methods) that you can live with for a few more months. You won't want to take your baby for a car ride every time he is sleepy or have to tread up and the down the stairs with an ever-heavier baby whenever he wakes in the middle of the night.

ALL THAT CRYING: SOME EXPLANATIONS

✳ Some people will tell you that babies cry only if they're cold or hungry or wet or sick. As you know by now, babies also cry when they're tired. But at this age, there are some other possible reasons for the tears:

Neurological development. Some crying may be stimulated by events that occur in your baby's brain at this age. Babies are born with a surplus of neurons (nerve cells); at this time, the baby's brain is in the dramatic and important process of trimming back some of those so-called excess neurons and neural pathways between cells. This pruning process allows the brain to become more efficient and focused. It also appears to allow the brain's newly emerging alertness mechanisms to surface. Alertness mechanisms help the baby become more aware of the world around him, but for reasons we don't yet understand, this adjustment or transition seems to be hard and especially distressing for some babies. Change is difficult for them, and crying is the only tool in the newborn baby's arsenal of coping techniques. Use the N.A.P.S. plan to give your child some much-needed rest during this tough time.

Sensory overload. Another reason for crying at this age is the sensory overload that babies experience. Imagine what the transition from womb to world must be like for them. They move from a dark and quiet place into a new environment, one with lots of sights, smells, sounds, and other sensations. The world's exciting sensory information is noise to babies. They can't make sense of this noise, and they can't get away from it. Worse, this noise keeps them from "hearing" the bodily signals for sleep.

THE WORLD'S EXCITING SENSORY INFORMATION IS NOISE TO BABIES. THEY CAN'T MAKE SENSE OF THIS NOISE, AND THEY CAN'T GET AWAY FROM IT. WORSE, THIS NOISE KEEPS THEM FROM "HEARING" THE BODILY SIGNALS FOR SLEEP.

That's where you come in. When you hear your baby cry, remember that he needs you to provide an unstimulating environment so sleep mechanisms can take over. Make things monotonous and nonalerting for your baby—with repetitive motions like rocking or songs that you sing over and over—so he can tune out the noisy, distracting world and sleep. Without any change to divert his attention, the unrelenting sameness of the repetition will help him disengage from his environment.

Evening fussiness. Evening fussiness is common in young babies. It usually starts at around two weeks of age and ends by the second or third month. Its timing can be strikingly consistent from night to night, coming on and winding down at predictable times. This period of crying can seem as if it will go on forever. I can recall feeling very discouraged and nearly despairing with my first child, Maddie, as the evening approached and she would crank up as if on cue and start to cry hard.

Some people attribute evening fussiness to colic or to parental exhaustion at the end of a long day, and those factors can indeed have a role in all that crying. But a more likely culprit is the emergence of circadian rhythms. In several studies of biological rhythms and the timing of sleep across a 24-hour period, adults show something called the "forbidden zone" for sleep. This is a period of time in the early evening when it's difficult for us to initiate sleep, no matter how tired we are. One theory is that a newborn baby's fussy period is nature's attempt to implant this feature in a baby's brain.

The best way to handle this difficult time is to reduce stimulation. Don't try to distract the baby with television, toys, or funny songs and faces. These tactics may briefly calm the baby, but don't be fooled. Soon the sensory stimulation will make the baby even more uncomfortable and upset. Accept that the baby will be fussy, and take whatever comfort you can in knowing that the crying is not caused by anything you have done. Evening fussiness is a developmental phase, and, thankfully, it is a temporary one. Instead, use your favorite method of comforting, repetitive soothing, and look to the N.A.P.S. plan as a guide for initiating sleep. When things seem bleak, remember that the baby's alertness window is never more than an hour and a half. Parents who ignore the 90-minute alertness cycle may find themselves with a baby who is not just dealing with the emergence of circadian rhythms but who is seriously overtired.

Colic. Colic is defined as inconsolable crying that occurs at predictable times of the day or night and cannot be explained by hunger, illness, discomfort, or other causes. It typically begins at around three weeks of age, and usually tapers off by the third or fourth month. Parents of colicky babies may say, "My baby cries for hours and hours" or even "My baby cries all the time."

The N.A.P.S. plan drastically reduces mysterious crying in most babies, including those who have been labeled colicky. Again and again, parents tell me how their baby's so-called colic went away or dramatically declined once they started using the program. I wonder whether these babies were truly colicky to begin with. I suspect that some babies with colic symptoms are simply very tired or are suffering from predictable evening fussiness.

But some babies cry a great deal even when they are well rested and when they are not in the throes of evening fussiness; in fact, these babies may seem to do nothing but cry, sleep, eat, and then cry some more. For parents of these truly colicky babies, I suggest following all the steps of the N.A.P.S. plan, with a few additional measures. Try setting a timer after the baby wakes up and then inducing sleep after 90 minutes; the timer will be necessary because the signs of sleepiness may be hard to spot against the backdrop of nearly constant crying. Rocking may not be enough for colicky children, so you can also try wearing the baby in a sling or front pack, or provide soothing repetitive sounds, such as a recording of the clothes dryer or vacuum cleaner running. Don't worry that these strategies will create bad sleep habits. You can wean your baby from them later, when you teach sleep

Jody's Story: *I'm Smiling*

"For the first two weeks after my daughter was born, I thought, 'What do new mothers have to complain about? This is so easy!' And then she became really colicky. She would cry for four hours every evening, wake up frequently at night, and fuss during the day. My mother was staying with me, and she'd say, 'Oh, the baby's tired.' But I kept her up during the day because I thought it would help her sleep at night. I had this beautiful, healthy baby, and I loved her—but I literally felt sick from lack of sleep, as if I were going to throw up.

"I decided to take four days to try the N.A.P.S. plan. I understood the idea of biorhythms and that an infant's attention span is only 90 minutes, and I liked the idea of giving my baby more sleep.

"The first time I tried the plan, I swaddled the baby and rocked her and made 'shhhh'ing sounds to comfort her—actually, I was doing this off and on for most of her alertness cycle because she was so fussy. At the end of 90 minutes, she was calm but not quite asleep. I put her down in the crib because my feet were cold and I wanted to get some socks. I left the room, thinking she would start to cry and I would need to get back quickly to help her. But when I returned, she was asleep. She slept for four hours.

"The colic ended almost as soon as I began following the N.A.P.S. plan, and nights got better. After eighty minutes, I would see her starting to get cranky. I used the same comforting techniques (swaddling, rocking, shushing) I'd tried before I knew about the 90-minute cycle, but now they actually worked—because I was following the baby's timing. The more I

> followed my baby's rhythm, the less it felt like she and I were fighting each other. She also started to feed better. Before, I had been feeding her all the time, but she'd eat for only five or seven minutes at a stretch. After she started taking longer naps, she began to eat for fifteen minutes at a time and had a chance to get full.
>
> "My baby and I started to bond again, like we did in the first two weeks. I feel happy as a mom again. She's smiling. I'm smiling!"

independence (see pages 94 to 101); for now, do what needs to be done. Don't feel guilty, because colic isn't your fault. And get as much help from your spouse, relatives, friends, or babysitters as you can until this difficult period is over.

YOUR BABY'S GOT (AN EMERGING) RHYTHM

✳ As you begin using the N.A.P.S. plan, you may not see a precise nap schedule materialize right away. That is, you may not see a morning nap at precisely 9:00 AM and an afternoon nap at 1:00 PM one day and then the next and the next. *Not at first.* Nap length at this age will vary, and your baby may have several long naps each day or maybe five or six naps of irregular duration. That's all right, because you are letting your baby's sleep patterns evolve on their own. This should pay off huge dividends later. And even though there is no hard-and-fast routine yet, by the end of this period your days will start to take on a rhythm, which most parents find a welcome change from the chaos of the early weeks. You'll enjoy looking forward to a nearly-90-minute period of playtime with your baby and also appreciate knowing that you'll soon have a break while the baby sleeps.

In the first three months, bedtime is often rather late. Many parents put their babies down around 10:00 PM or so, for example. Night wakings may still occur at this age, and they are normal, but the N.A.P.S. plan can help minimize them, by producing a well-rested baby who is more able to make a smooth transition from one complete sleep cycle to another.

In time, as your baby matures and the sleep rhythms develop, short naps will stretch into longer ones, bedtime will start earlier, the number of night wakings will decrease, and your baby will start to follow a schedule.

DAY/NIGHT CONFUSION: GOOD NEWS

✳ Just as the 90-minute clocks are being established during this period, circadian (daily) rhythms also emerge. These 24-hour rhythms are usually established by the 46th week after conception or about six weeks after birth for a full-term baby. As I described earlier, circadian rhythms can cause evening fussiness. However, their appearance is actually good news for you because they will help your baby move his longest sleep bout of the 24-hour period to the night—where it most definitely belongs! Until then, keep up the good habits of using dim light (or red light) and a quiet voice when your baby is awake in the night. When you discover that your baby is wide awake at 2:00 or 3:00 AM, and you are unable to comfort or feed him back to sleep, don't despair. There's no good reason a young baby should be awake any longer than 90 minutes. This is true even at night, and it is true even if the baby took

NAP MAPS FOR EIGHT-WEEK-OLD BABIES

To show you how nap patterns emerge, here are "nap maps" for three young babies: Mia, Jack, and Isaac. Each baby is eight weeks old, and each set of parents is committed to helping their child follow his or her internal rhythms. At this young age, nap length varies, and so do the number of naps, so every baby's day will look different and will probably change from one day to another. (Older babies usually develop more predictable schedules, often somewhere between three and six months.) These are *nap* maps, so aside from bedtime and wake-up time, information about night sleep is not included. *Don't try to make your baby follow any of these schedules.* They are just sample days to help you see how the program works.

Notice that the interval between each awakening and the subsequent sleep period is consistently 90 minutes, no matter how long or short the nap. Throughout this chapter and the next, we'll follow Mia, Jack, and Isaac as they grow older and their nap patterns change.

MIA'S NAPS	JACK'S NAPS	ISAAC'S NAPS
Wake-up	Wake-up	Wake-up
5:30 AM	7:30 AM	6:45 AM
First nap	First nap	First nap
7:00 AM–8:30 AM	9:00 AM–9:20 AM	8:15 AM–10:45 AM
Second nap	Second nap	Second nap
10:00 AM–11:30 AM	10:50 AM–1:50 PM	12:15 PM–3:15 PM
Third nap	Third nap	Third nap
1:00 PM–4:00 PM	3:20 PM–4:00 PM	4:45 PM–7:45 PM
Fourth nap	Fourth nap	Bedtime
5:30 PM–6:00 PM	5:30 PM–6:00 PM	9:15 PM
Fifth nap	Fifth nap	
7:30 PM–9:00 PM	7:30 PM–9:30 PM	
Bedtime	Bedtime	
10:30 PM	11:00 PM	

a very long nap the previous day. Once you realize this, you won't need to panic when your baby wakes up at 3:00 AM, bright and playful. In the worst-case scenario, he will be back asleep by 4:30 AM. (Remember

Jennifer's Story: *My Husband Thought I Was Crazy*

"My daughter, Ada, has always been a good night sleeper, even from a very young age. But she did not nap well during the day at all. I had trouble accepting the N.A.P.S. plan at first. It was counterintuitive that after sleeping for 11 hours at night, Ada would need to go down for another nap in the early morning.

"But I started putting her down to sleep 90 minutes after she woke up in the morning, and that worked. She really needed the sleep; she started getting fussy if she didn't get it. My husband thought I was crazy until he saw how it worked.

"One problem we've had is that there is a lot of pressure now to take your baby out with you everywhere, to continue your life with your newborn baby along. I don't think people had this issue ten or fifteen years ago. You're supposed to go to lunches and parties and go shopping and just bring your baby along with you. Other parents we know have babies who sleep in infant seats and travel gear. A few of them seem to get nice long naps even when they're parked in their strollers. But my baby has never been very good at sleeping in public. She really needed to be helped to sleep even in the first weeks. It isn't always easy to resist the social calendars, but I know that one of the reasons I'm staying at home these early months is to adapt to my baby's needs."

not to encourage playtime in the middle of the night; even while your baby is awake, keep things quiet and dark. If you need to pick him up, fine—just don't haul out the whirring toys and turn on all the lights.) Simply knowing there is an end in sight can help you cope.

THE N.A.P.S. PLAN AT A GLANCE

Two Weeks to Three Months

- The 90-minute cycle will take effect during this period if it hasn't already. Use the N.A.P.S. plan to ensure that your baby gets sufficient sleep.

- Most babies of this age need approximately fifteen to sixteen hours of sleep daily.

- You may not see a regular nap schedule yet, but your days and nights will become more rhythmic if you follow the N.A.P.S. plan.

- Mysterious fussing is often a sign that your baby is tired. It may also be caused by neurological development, colic, or evening fussiness. The N.A.P.S. plan should help, but if you're concerned that the fussiness might be a sign of a

medical condition, consult your pediatrician.

- At this age, most babies still need your help to get to sleep.

- Continue to give your baby a chance to settle back down to sleep if he opens his eyes or makes noises without crying.

- Day/night confusion often reverses itself by week eight, if not before. Until then, remember that your baby should not be awake at night for more than 90 minutes at a time.

- During this period, your baby may lose his ability to fall asleep and stay asleep during outings. If this happens, try to structure your days so you are at home for baby's nap times.

Three Through Five Months

As your baby exits the newborn period, life becomes calmer. Most babies cry less, and their parents feel more confident and start to enjoy their babies more. It's a delight to see glimmers of your baby's personality as he has fun exploring his world. But it's probably been a long three months, and any reserves of energy you'd saved up before the baby arrived may now be running low. You still need to rest when you can and accept—or solicit—offers of help from family and friends.

> **YOU STILL NEED TO REST WHEN YOU CAN AND ACCEPT—OR SOLICIT—OFFERS OF HELP FROM FAMILY AND FRIENDS.**

At this age, your baby needs around fourteen or fifteen hours of sleep per day. Most of this sleep should occur during the nighttime hours, although you'll still see frequent naps throughout the day. As you'll learn, some important changes occur in the three-month to six-month-birthday period. Naps start to lengthen and become more consistent; bedtime moves earlier in the evening; and the length of some wakeful cycles may double or even triple.

NAP LENGTH AND CONSISTENCY

✳ Between three months and the six-month birthday, babies start to consolidate their short, frequent naps into fewer and longer daytime sleep periods. Usually, parents see the emergence of three naps at this time: one in the morning, one in the afternoon, and one in the late afternoon or early evening. The evening nap is often very short. If your child needs an evening nap, give it to him. An evening nap does not interfere with good nighttime sleep in babies.

Don't worry if your baby doesn't follow this three-nap pattern! Some babies need fewer or more naps during the day depending on how much sleep they get at night and the length of their naps. Some babies take just two naps, provided their naps are long and they go to bed early. Other babies need four naps, and still others continue to take several short, frequent naps at this age. If your baby is a catnapper, continue to put him down toward the end of the 90-minute cycle, even if this results in five or six naps daily. If the naps don't lengthen on their own by the time he is six months old, you can take steps to improve them (see pages 127 to 129).

No matter how many naps your baby takes, the length and timing of those naps should start to become somewhat predictable from day to day. The N.A.P.S. plan promotes this consistency.

BEDTIME

✳ By the time babies are four or five months old, most no longer naturally stay up late in the evening; their bedtimes begin to shift much earlier. Most babies who are this age and older prefer a bedtime that occurs between 6:00 PM and 8:00 PM. I caution parents who work outside the home to resist the temptation to keep their babies up late. Most babies (and toddlers—consider yourself warned!) wake up early in the morning when the sky first brightens, and even after a late bedtime they are often unable to sleep later in the morning to make up the missed sleep.

Even when it's possible to keep a baby up late and postpone the morning wake-up time, I discourage the practice. It's important for a baby's developing brain to register the rising of the sun. This is a significant cue for the brain's clocks, which regulate much more of our physiology than just sleep and waking. Many of our body processes are optimized when they are synchronized with body clocks. You can ask anyone who works the night shift about this phenomenon. People on the night shift tend not to be terribly alert during their work hours and have trouble sleeping when they're off. They have significantly higher rates of certain diseases, and their life expectancy is shorter. When I encounter parents who are determined to alter an early bedtime, I remind them that sleep is a basic biological need. Although at certain times a later bedtime is necessary, do your very best to let your baby turn in early, even if it means you get less time with him at night. Maybe you can find time in the early morning to have fun with your child; most babies are happiest and most receptive at this time anyway.

 IT'S IMPORTANT FOR A BABY'S DEVELOPING BRAIN TO REGISTER THE RISING OF THE SUN. THIS IS A SIGNIFICANT CUE FOR THE BRAIN'S CLOCKS, WHICH REGULATE MUCH MORE OF OUR PHYSIOLOGY THAN JUST SLEEP AND WAKING.

EXTENDED PLAYTIME

✳ There is no single precise age at which babies become capable of staying awake for longer than 90 minutes. Sometime after the fourth month or so, however, many babies extend one or more of their wakeful cycles from 90 minutes to three hours (which is two consecutive 90-minute cycles) or even four and a half hours (which is three consecutive 90-minute cycles). No matter when your baby begins to stay awake for longer periods, there are some fairly predictable ways this change takes shape. The first longer wakeful period usually appears in the evening, just before bedtime. It can also appear just after the morning awakening. Although you might expect this change to occur in gradual increments, from 90 minutes of wakefulness to 100 minutes to 110 minutes and so on, babies usually make the transition rather suddenly, from 90 minutes straight to 180 or 270 minutes.

How do you know if your baby is ready to extend one of his wakeful cycles? Every baby follows the dictates of his inner schedule, so you'll have to follow your child's cues, not an external timetable. I remember being surprised when my daughter stopped falling asleep at her customary evening nap times. She wasn't particularly fussy in the crib, just contentedly wakeful. I also noticed that she remained cheerful until bedtime 90 minutes later. These were my clues! After a few evenings of this behavior, I realized she had dropped her short evening nap and moved on to a longer wakeful cycle in the evening.

If your child starts to extend her morning wakeful period, her first nap of the day may become shorter. For example, if your child's morning schedule currently looks like this:

Wake-up: 6:30 AM

Morning nap: 8:00 AM–11:00 AM

It may soon look like this:

Wake-up: 6:30 AM

Morning nap: 9:30 AM–11:00 AM

Don't be fooled into thinking that the morning nap has disappeared! It is merely shorter. Your baby will probably continue to follow a 90-minute cycle for the rest of the day, perhaps with a longer wakeful period just before bedtime. As always, don't force your baby into longer periods of wakefulness. Watch your child's cues, which will tell you when your child is ready to sleep.

Some babies seem to adopt longer alertness periods—whether in the evening, in the morning, or both—virtually overnight. Other babies spend a few days or weeks making the transition. They may want long wakeful periods on some days but not on others. You'll need to summon your patience until the transition is complete, because your baby may be extra tired on the days he doesn't nap as much. Soon enough, you'll both adjust to the new routine. You may miss the extra rest time, but you'll also enjoy having longer intervals when you don't have to think about the baby's naps.

NIGHT WAKINGS: FEED OR SOOTHE?

∗ Parents who read books and take classes before the baby is born are given a great deal of information about feeding their babies. That's good, because feeding a newborn can be harder than it looks. In the early weeks and months, babies are hungry at frequent and irregular intervals, and they should be fed on demand. Unfortunately, though, experts sometimes focus solely on hunger as a reason for night wakings, making it easy to overlook other possible reasons a baby wakes up at night.

We tend to think that food is the primary organizing force of a baby's life and that babies *always* awaken out of hunger at night and therefore must be fed at each waking. Although babies do awaken from hunger, sometimes the cause of the wakings is the immature state of a baby's

NAP MAPS FOR FIVE-MONTH-OLD BABIES

S everal changes take place between three months and the six-month birthday: Consistent nap patterns develop; bedtime moves earlier; and longer wakeful periods (in increments of 90 minutes) may develop, especially in the evening. Here are some sample schedules that show you how these changes may take hold. Remember that your baby will probably not follow any of these schedules to the letter. Instead, your baby will develop his own schedule.

MIA'S NAPS

Mia has started to take three regular naps: two naps in the morning and afternoon, and one short nap just before dinner. She has developed a three-hour wakeful period after waking up and in the early evening. and her bedtime has moved to 8:00 PM.

Wake-up
7:00 AM

Morning nap
10:00 AM–11:30 AM

Afternoon nap
1:00 PM–3:00 PM

Late afternoon nap
4:30 PM–5:00 PM

Bedtime
8:00 PM

JACK'S NAPS

Jack now takes a series of fairly short naps throughout the day. His parents are thankful that he goes to bed early! Jack does not yet have any long wakeful periods, a pattern that is common in babies who take short naps.

Wake-up
6:00 AM

First nap
7:30 AM–8:30 AM

Second nap
10:00 AM–11:00 AM

Third nap
12:30 PM–1:00 PM

Fourth nap
2:30 PM–3:00 PM

Fifth nap
4:30 PM–5:00 PM

Bedtime
6:30 PM

ISAAC'S NAPS

Isaac takes two very long naps during the day. He has 90-minute wakeful cycles during the day, except for a four-and-a-half-hour wakeful period in the evening.

Wake-up
6:30 AM

First nap
8:00 AM–11:00 AM

Second nap
2:00 PM–4:00 PM

Bedtime
8:30 PM

nervous system, and sometimes the cause is insufficient daytime sleep. If your baby isn't genuinely hungry at night and you feed him anyway, two problems are created. The first is that you haven't addressed the real issue, which is that the baby wants to be comforted back to sleep. The second is that you may have unintentionally trained your baby to awaken at the same time in the nights to come. Feedings are remarkably strong cues for nighttime awakenings. Experimental animals presented with food during a sleep period quickly learn to awaken at the same time the next day or night and look for a snack.

Of course, this all sounds fine in theory, but in real life it can be hard for parents to know what to do. The trouble is that when your baby cries at night, you can't know with certainty why he's upset. Is he hungry or just longing to return to sleep? In the middle of the night, feeding is the simplest solution: The baby stops crying, and often the baby falls back to sleep.

Before you try to reduce nighttime feedings, check with your pediatrician. If your baby has trouble gaining weight or has other health problems, feeding may in fact be the most appropriate response at each waking. If that's the case, follow your doctor's advice. Even if your baby is gaining weight and is healthy, recognize that in the first few months, your baby is probably truly hungry much of the time.

After the newborn period, however, most parents can read their baby's cries and determine from their sound whether the baby is hungry, uncomfortable, bored, or sleepy. Listen for these cues before automatically assuming that your baby is hungry, and give him a chance to tell you what he needs. If you have fed him recently, and if he awakens at the end of a sleep cycle (say, at the end of 90 minutes, three hours, four and a half hours, six hours, or any other multiple of the 90-minute cycle), try soothing him back to sleep by rocking or walking, or patting him as he lies in his crib, instead of immediately offering food. If this doesn't work, you can try feeding him.

Data back up this nighttime strategy. In a 1993 study published in the journal *Pediatrics,* a group of mothers were told to feed their newborn babies whenever the babies awoke crying in the night. Another group was told to give their babies a "focal feeding" between 10:00 PM and midnight; if the babies woke up later in the night, they were to try to stretch out the intervals between feedings by using alternative comforting strategies whenever possible, although they could certainly feed their babies if the babies seemed hungry. Eight weeks later, *all* of the babies whose mothers used alternative soothing strategies were now sleeping for at least five hours straight—specifically, between midnight and 5:00 AM. Fewer than 25 percent of the babies in the feeding group had accomplished this feat. This study also discovered that babies in both groups were ingesting the same quantity of food over a 24-hour period.

EIGHT WEEKS LATER, ALL OF THE BABIES WHOSE MOTHERS USED ALTERNATIVE SOOTHING STRATEGIES WERE NOW SLEEPING FOR AT LEAST FIVE HOURS STRAIGHT— SPECIFICALLY, BETWEEN MIDNIGHT AND 5:00 AM. FEWER THAN 25 PERCENT OF THE BABIES IN THE FEEDING GROUP HAD ACCOMPLISHED THIS FEAT.

This study is good news for breastfeeding mothers. I am a strong supporter of breastfeeding and am troubled when mothers are told that breast milk is thinner or less adequate than formula and thus less likely to "stay in the baby's stomach." This assumption often leads mothers to give up on breastfeeding for the dubious sleep benefits of the bottle. Others put their baby to the breast frequently at night in the belief that their baby needs a constant supply of breast milk to stay nourished. In fact, this study suggests that if mothers do not rely solely on feedings during night wakings, the babies make up the calories elsewhere in the day, and they learn to sleep through the night earlier.

IF IT'S POSSIBLE FOR YOU SIMPLY TO HOLD YOUR YOUNG BABY AND ROCK HIM BACK TO SLEEP, YOU'VE TAUGHT HIM A POWERFUL LESSON AND AVOIDED MAKING A CONNECTION BETWEEN FATIGUE AND FOOD.

I want to stress again that you never want to deprive a hungry baby or avoid feeding a baby who has trouble gaining weight. But if it's possible for you simply to hold your young baby and rock him back to sleep, you've taught him a powerful lesson and avoided making a connection between fatigue and food.

As your baby grows older, and with your pediatrician's blessing, you can also stretch out the interval between daytime feedings, which has a positive effect on night sleep. Aim for four hours between feedings by six months, if you can—if earlier than that, great. Babies who are fed every two hours in the day often wake up repeatedly at night, possibly because they are conditioned to expect frequent feedings and thus awaken to get them.

THREE MYTHS ABOUT FOOD AND SLEEP

Do heavier babies sleep better? Will rice cereal help a baby sleep for longer stretches? Let's look at some common myths about food and infant sleep.

MYTH *Babies need to weigh twelve (or nine, or fourteen) pounds before they can sleep through the night.*

Studies fail to bear out the theory that babies need to weigh a certain amount before they can go through the night. I've certainly seen quite a few upper-weight babies who are unable to sleep well. Yet some people continue to believe in one of these magic numbers. Age is actually a better indicator of a baby's readiness to sleep through the night because age, not weight, more closely reflects neural development. As a general rule (and there are exceptions), most normally developing and growing babies should no longer need night feedings by the age of six months.

MYTH *Breastfeeding causes babies to wake up more often.*

I would never encourage a mother to discontinue breastfeeding in the hopes that her baby will sleep for longer periods. First and foremost, the benefits of breastfeeding are too well documented to ignore. And although some studies show that bottle-fed babies sleep for longer stretches at night than breastfed babies do, other studies come to the opposite conclusion. Few of the studies take into account whether a baby gets sufficient daytime sleep. However, if a mother relies solely on putting the baby to the breast as a way to help the baby back to sleep, the baby can become conditioned to expect feedings several times a night—and he will wake up to get them.

MYTH *Solid food helps babies sleep longer.*

You may have heard that your baby will sleep for longer periods at night if you start feeding him rice cereal. Perhaps this is true for a few individual babies, but not for all. Rice cereal (or other solids) does not always extend sleep length in infants. It makes me sad when parents are assured that cereal is a kind of guaranteed sleep food and then blame themselves (or the baby) when it doesn't work. Worse, putting rice cereal in a baby's bottle can lead to rapid and unhealthy weight gain.

Here's the bottom line: Don't look to food as a guaranteed way to help your baby sleep through the night. Instead, work on good nap habits during the day, and remember that babies can wake up at night for reasons other than hunger.

SELF-SOOTHING: MAKE A TRIAL RUN

✳ Although self-soothing techniques work better on older babies, a few babies in the three-month to six-month-birthday age bracket are able to fall asleep on their own, especially if they have been on the N.A.P.S. plan and have started to make a connection between fatigue and the need to sleep. You can try soothing your baby at the end of the 90-minute cycle and then putting him down while he is drowsy but still awake; possibly he will close his eyes and drift off without any further intervention from you.

MANY BABIES AREN'T READY TO FALL ASLEEP INDEPENDENTLY UNTIL THEY ARE AROUND SIX MONTHS OLD; SOME BABIES, A LITTLE LATER THAN THAT.

If he fusses a little, you can pat him or sing to him to see if he can settle down. But if the baby starts up a full-blown wail, he's probably not ready yet for self-soothing. Pick him up and continue your usual soothing routine until he is asleep. You can try again when he's a little older. Many babies aren't ready to fall asleep independently until they are around six months old; some babies, a little later than that (see pages 94 to 101 for more on self-soothing).

You might also consider the pick-up/put-down method, a no-cry strategy popularized by Traci Hogg in her *Baby Whisperer* books. Its premise is simple: Soothe the baby until he is drowsy. Put him in the crib while he is still awake. If he cries, pick him up and soothe him until he is quietly sleepy again. Then put him down. Continue this pattern of picking the baby up, soothing him, and putting him back down until he either falls asleep in the crib or until his playfulness tells you that he has entered another alertness cycle. The pick-up/put-down method works well for some babies but is confusing or stimulating for many others. It's painless, however, so it's worth a try.

Beware that babies who are temperamentally more difficult, more social, or who are not well rested have a harder time falling asleep on their own. And timing is crucial: A baby who is put down in the middle of his alertness cycle will not fall asleep, no matter how exhausted he may be. Wait until the end of the cycle when he is tired and ready to nod off. You may also find that your baby learns self-soothing more easily at bedtime than at naps.

THE N.A.P.S. PLAN AT A GLANCE

Three Through Five Months

- Most babies still require about fourteen or fifteen hours of sleep per day, although your baby may need more or less. By this age, babies who follow the N.A.P.S. plan should be getting a consistent amount of sleep from day to day.

- Continue the N.A.P.S. plan. This will encourage longer sleep periods during both day and night.

- By months four or five, bedtime moves earlier and you will probably see naps consolidate into predictable sleep periods. Many babies take a morning nap, an afternoon nap, and an evening nap, but don't worry if your baby needs more naps or fewer.

- Your baby may also develop the ability to stay awake for longer periods (usually lasting three hours or four and a half hours) during the day.

- If your baby wakes frequently at night, consider that he may not be hungry at each waking. After you have checked with your pediatrician—and *only* when you have received the doctor's approval—try to soothe your baby back to sleep without feeding him.

- Also ask your pediatrician if you can nudge the duration between daytime feedings farther apart, so the interval between feedings is about four hours. Know that some babies have health issues that require more frequent feedings.

- At the end of an alertness cycle, try putting your baby down when she is drowsy but awake. Your baby may surprise you by falling asleep without protest. Don't be alarmed if she doesn't. It's still too early for many babies to soothe themselves to sleep.

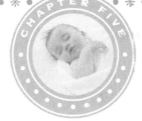

CHAPTER FIVE

The N.A.P.S. Plan
Six Months to One Year and Beyond

I n the second half of the first year of life, babies reach a new level of neurological maturity, and parents have a greater chance of getting some of their old life back. This is because older babies are more capable of falling asleep on their own, sleeping through the night, increasing their alertness windows, and developing a schedule.

Six to Eight Months

When your baby reaches the six-month milestone, she will still need plenty of sleep—usually between thirteen and fourteen hours daily. Keep up her good sleep habits by continuing the N.A.P.S. plan. You'll have some adjustments to make as the baby further extends her wakeful periods and possibly learns to fall asleep on her own, but if your baby is well rested, these transitions should be fairly smooth. If your baby is still taking short, frequent naps or is waking up often at night, don't despair. The baby is now old enough to learn a few sleep skills, and this section will show you how to teach them.

WATCH FOR ANOTHER LONG WAKEFUL PERIOD

✳ Your baby may already be able to stay awake for three or four and a half hours at certain times of the day, especially in the evening or after waking up in the morning. Now you can expect yet another three-hour wakeful period to emerge sometime after the six-month birthday, although in a few babies it won't appear until seven, eight, or nine months of age. It usually occurs between the morning and afternoon naps.

HELPING YOUR BABY FALL ASLEEP ON HER OWN

✳ Here's one of the questions I am most frequently asked: How do I get my baby to fall asleep on her own? In the first months of life, most babies aren't capable of falling asleep without assistance because they can't shut out the noise of the world. Up to this point, you have probably been rocking the baby, lying down with her, or perhaps nursing her until she is soundly asleep. (I don't advocate nursing babies to sleep after they are past the newborn stage, but some parents find that this is the only technique that works, especially if the baby is colicky.)

But the period between six and eight months provides a golden opportunity. For one thing, although it can sometimes be tough to teach your baby self-soothing, it's generally as easy at this age as it's ever going to be. This is when babies are neurologically ready to fall

Nap Maps for Seven-Month-Old Babies

Around this age you may see the emergence of another alertness period, but keep in mind that babies follow their own timetable—this period will develop in your own baby when he or she is ready. Remember, too, that the schedules outlined below are only samples, not timelines that your baby must adhere to. Try to let your baby's routine evolve naturally.

Mia's Naps

Mia's day remains the same as it did at five months of age (see page 85). She has not yet extended the time between her naps or dropped her evening nap, and her parents should not pressure her to do so.

Wake-up
7:00 AM

Morning nap
10:00 AM–11:30 AM

Afternoon nap
1:00 PM–3:00 PM

Late afternoon nap
4:30 PM–5:00 PM

Bedtime
8:00 PM

Jack's Naps

Jack's schedule has changed quite a bit since he was five months old and took five short naps a day (see page 85). His parents used the self-soothing techniques described on pages 98 to 101 to help Jack extend his naps, and now he takes two naps daily. Jack has also developed three periods of extended wakefulness: one in the morning, one between naps, and one before bed.

Wake-up
6:00 AM

First nap
9:00 AM–11:00 AM

Second nap
2:00 PM–3:00 PM

Bedtime
7:30 PM

Isaac's Naps

When Isaac was five months old, he was taking only two long naps daily, with no evening nap (see page 85). At seven months, Isaac's pattern remains similar, except that he stays awake longer in the morning, his first nap is shorter, and he stays awake for three hours between naps.

Wake-up
6:30 AM

First nap
9:30 AM–11:00 AM

Second nap
2:00 PM–3:30 PM

Bedtime
8:00 PM

asleep independently, but psychologically they are still flexible and not yet strongly attached to particular sleep habits. Later on, it's still possible but is often more difficult.

Teaching babies to soothe themselves brings several rewards:

1. A baby who learns to fall asleep on her own will usually start to sleep through the night shortly thereafter.

2. Self-soothing helps the baby take longer naps.

3. Putting the baby to bed will become an enjoyable ritual, not an emotionally and physically draining process.

4. Your baby learns self-sufficiency, a valuable skill.

If your baby falls asleep easily in your arms or while nursing, you may be tempted to put off teaching self-soothing techniques indefinitely. Or you may outwardly complain about the baby's dependence at nighttime but secretly enjoy it. It's natural to appreciate being indispensable and needed. These feelings are understandable, but be careful. Parents who miss the window of opportunity for self-soothing can later wind up with a toddler who depends on their presence to sleep. As the child grows older, this dependence can turn into bedtime power struggles.

> **THERE IS NO SINGLE "RIGHT" WAY TO TEACH SELF-SOOTHING SKILLS, NO MATTER WHAT ANYONE TELLS YOU. THE BEST METHOD IS THE ONE THAT FITS YOUR BABY'S PERSONALITY AND ALLOWS HER TO FALL ASLEEP ACCORDING TO HER INNER RHYTHMS.**

There is no single "right" way to teach self-soothing skills, no matter what anyone tells you. The best method is the one that fits your baby's personality *and* allows her to fall asleep according to her inner rhythms. Before you start teaching sleep independence, here are a few preliminary things you can do to increase your chances of success:

Establish a bedtime routine. Set up a brief series of comforting activities, such as a short warm bath followed by a book or a lullaby. Make sure that you can easily repeat these activities before bedtime each night. Soon your baby will associate these events with going to sleep. If your baby needs to be nursed or otherwise soothed to sleep, continue to do so for now. Make sure the final element of the routine occurs in the baby's room and that bedtime occurs at the end of the alertness cycle. Don't let your dread about bedtime make you turn the routine into a long drawn-out process. In the months and years to come, you'll be glad you didn't.

Make sure that your child is well rested. Giving a crash course in self-soothing to someone who is sleep deprived seems cruel and unusual to me. Think about how you feel when you are sleep deprived: At these times, what's your attitude to a sudden change? Not so good, I'll bet. Often people think, "The baby is so tired that she'll drop right off and she won't protest at all." These are famous last words! Exhaustion doesn't make self-soothing easier; in fact, the process can backfire— and backfire badly—when a baby is sleep deprived.

If your baby has not been on the N.A.P.S. plan and is overtired, set aside a few days to start N.A.P.S. and make sure the baby gets all the sleep she needs. If the only way your baby can get a decent amount of sleep is for you to drive her around in the car for naps, or wear her in a sling or front pack, or put her in a mechanical swing, do it—for now. Once your baby is getting more sleep and you have a notion about the general timing of her naps, you can move the baby to a crib and initiate sleep training.

Clear your schedule and check with the neighbors. Don't attempt to teach your baby self-soothing when you know that the household sleep routine will soon be disrupted by overnight guests or a vacation. Avoid using self-soothing techniques during times of major change for your baby—weaning, a parent going back to work, the birth of a sibling, or a move to a new house. If you live in an apartment building where the walls or floors are thin, talk to your neighbors. Explain what you are doing and let them know that they may hear some crying. Come up with a time that's convenient for everyone—and not when your neighbors are planning to throw a loud party.

Next I've listed two choices for teaching your baby sleep independence while following the 90-minute cycle. I suggest you begin at bedtime, teaching the baby to fall asleep on her own when she goes down for the night, rather than at nap time. Within a few days or weeks the positive results are likely to generalize themselves to night wakings and to daytime naps. Evenings are also when both parents are likely to be home, and it's helpful to have your spouse around for emotional support.

Self-soothing technique #1: Controlled crying. Also known as "crying it out," this is one of the fastest methods of teaching your baby to self-soothe and is backed by the most research on its effectiveness. Begin by following

ALSO KNOWN AS "CRYING IT OUT," THIS IS ONE OF THE FASTEST METHODS OF TEACHING YOUR BABY TO SELF-SOOTHE.

the N.A.P.S. plan all day, helping your baby sleep as you normally would, even if you use a sling or put the baby down sound asleep. At night, go through your bedtime routine, timing the activities so your baby is ready for bed at the end of her alertness cycle. Perform your usual soothing method, but stop while she is drowsy and not yet asleep. Place her in the crib, kiss her goodnight, and leave the room.

Now comes the hard part! The baby may protest this change in routine by crying, but you should not go to her right away. Instead, wait five minutes or so. If she doesn't settle down on her own, go into her room. Pat her and reassure her, but don't pick her up. Don't spend more than a minute with her before you leave the room again. Continue this pattern of waiting five minutes and then checking on the baby. If you sense that your baby is stimulated by these check-in periods or if she seems to be winding down and preparing to sleep, by all means follow your instincts and stay out for a longer time.

Controlled crying sometimes gets a bad reputation from parents whose children are chronically tired and unaccustomed to heeding their body's sleep signals. These kids can take hours to fall asleep on their own. But if you are following the N.A.P.S. plan, expect the process to involve much, *much* less crying—about fifteen minutes or so.

Despite the minimal amount of crying involved, this method is hard for some parents to bear. Its advantage is speed: When it works, it usually takes only three nights before the baby knows how to settle herself down for the evening. The first night can be tough, and the

IT USUALLY TAKES ONLY THREE NIGHTS BEFORE THE BABY KNOWS HOW TO SETTLE HERSELF DOWN FOR THE EVENING.

second night, when your baby may test you with a longer period of crying, can be even tougher. But by the third night, the process is usually complete.

What if fifteen minutes have passed and your baby is still crying? Some experts argue that it's wrong to put a time limit on the process because the baby will learn that you will rescue her if she cries long and hard enough. But most parents feel that crying that goes on for a very long time is unfair to the baby. It's also true that if your baby is awake and crying for more than fifteen minutes, she may enter another alertness cycle and be unable to fall asleep for the next 90 minutes. My advice for most parents is to go in after fifteen minutes of crying, pick the baby up, and try again at another date, perhaps in a few weeks. However, you know your baby better than anyone else. If you feel that she will wind down if she's given a little more time alone in the crib, you may well be right.

At other times you might need to call sleep training to a halt. You'll know the technique is too hard for your baby if the crying becomes more intense and distressed over time instead of more subdued. Some babies have a slightly later window of opportunity for learning self-soothing; you may have more success when they are older. Other babies who are temperamentally difficult or highly sociable may have a lower tolerance for being left alone (see page 124). A more gradual approach, which I describe next, may be more effective with them. Again, it's more important to match the self-soothing technique to your baby's personality and temperament than to your own preferences.

Self-soothing technique #2: Fading. Fading is a more gradual technique than controlled crying. It isn't as fast or reliable, but it minimizes the distress for some babies (and their parents!). The fading technique takes the baby from maximum parental presence to minimum parental presence over the course of several nights.

Begin with your established bedtime routine. At the end of the wakefulness cycle, perform your usual soothing method, but stop before the baby is asleep. Put the baby down in the crib and stay with her, patting her back or singing to her. She may protest by fussing or crying, but stay firm and do not pick her up. Continue this patting or singing routine for a few nights, until she is falling asleep easily. Once she is accustomed to falling asleep in the crib and not in your arms, you can simply sit in a nearby chair without touching or singing. A few nights later, move your chair farther away from the crib. Later, you can just stand in the doorway, so your child can see you but is much less dependent on your presence for sleep. Finally, you should reach a point where you can leave the room before the baby is asleep, and she will drift off by herself.

This procedure may appear to be much easier than controlled crying, at least in the sense that there are usually fewer tears, and for some babies and parents it *is* easier. For others, the process takes too long—sometimes days, sometimes weeks—and wears everyone out. Sometimes an interruption arrives in the form of illness or a business trip before the training period is over. Some babies actually have an easier time settling down when they are left alone in their familiar sleeping environment. For them, having the parent nearby but inaccessible is a source of agitation, not comfort.

CO-SLEEPING: MAKE SURE IT'S YOUR CHOICE

✳ If you are committed to co-sleeping with your children and do not wish to teach them self-soothing, embrace the experience and enjoy it—as long as you are fully informed about your choice.

Although co-sleeping can be a warm and snuggly experience with a little baby, be aware that things can change! Angelic little ones have a way of growing into toddlers who will thrash around in their sleep, wake up for middle-of-the-night play sessions, fall back asleep while lying horizontally across your bed, and generally make it extremely difficult for anyone to get a good night's rest. Many studies show that all members of co-sleeping families get less and poorer-quality sleep than those in which the children sleep in their own cribs or beds. Also keep in mind that teaching a six-month-old baby to sleep independently is *much* easier than teaching a four-year-old the same skill.

If you know about these drawbacks and still like the idea of co-sleeping, that's fine. But if your only reason for co-sleeping is that you're afraid your child will protest for hours if placed in a crib to sleep, I have some good news for you. Children on the N.A.P.S. plan often learn to sleep on their own after just a few minutes of protesting. Some learn without any crying at all. Why not give it a try? Self-soothing not only maximizes good sleep, it teaches your child self-efficacy. Both are life-long gifts to give your child.

SLEEPING THROUGH THE NIGHT

✳ "Sleeping through the night" is an inaccurate phrase. For one thing, there may be a dozen different ways to define what it is. For another thing, time-lapse video recordings and other forms of sleep monitoring show that all babies—even those identified as so-called good sleepers— wake up several times at night. These wakings usually occur at the end of REM periods. We all have these wakings, even if we don't recall them when we arise the next morning. In teaching babies to sleep well, we aren't teaching them to avoid waking up at night. We're teaching them how to go back to sleep on their own when they do.

These normal night stirrings can be alarming to a baby who has fallen asleep in your arms and then "suddenly" finds herself in a crib. This surprise is just the kind of thing that can bring a stirring baby to full alertness. "Hey!" she thinks. "What happened? Where'd you go, Mom?" She is now wide awake and needs you to comfort her until she returns to sleep. That's why it's so important to teach your baby how to fall asleep on her own. When babies learn how to fall asleep in their cribs at bedtime, they are much less disturbed during night wakings. "Oh," they think, in their half-awake state, "Here I am in my usual cozy spot. Think I'll close my eyes again." And usually in less than a minute, they are sound asleep.

If your baby is not yet sleeping through the night, your first step is to teach her how to fall asleep by herself at bedtime. You can continue to respond to her in your usual manner—nursing, rocking, or taking her into bed with you—if she wakes at night. Within a few weeks of learning to fall asleep on her own at the beginning of the night, she'll probably start to settle back to sleep on her own in the middle of the night.

If that doesn't happen, there are a few things you can do. Are you still feeding the baby at night? As I've described before, food is a powerful cue for waking. Try gradually withdrawing the food (by nursing for fewer minutes or putting less formula in the bottle) over a series of nights and then using alternative soothing techniques such as rocking to help the baby back to sleep. The overwhelming majority of babies who can fall asleep on their own at bedtime and who are not fed in the middle of the night start to sleep through until morning.

A few babies, however, continue to cry out for their parents. At this point, you can apply the controlled-crying or fading techniques to the night wakings. Or perhaps you'll find that although your baby cries once or twice at night, she will return to sleep after a very quick intervention from you, such as a few minutes of patting or rocking. If these

THE N.A.P.S. PLAN AT A GLANCE

Six to Eight Months

- Average sleep amounts for babies of this age are thirteen to fourteen hours daily. Your baby may need a little more or a little less.

- Continue to follow the N.A.P.S. plan. You may have already seen your baby develop longer periods of wakefulness in the evening and/or the morning; now your baby may also show a three-hour window of alertness between naps.

- Between six and eight months of age, most babies are ready to learn to fall asleep by themselves. Perform one of the self-soothing techniques described on pages 98 to 101 to take advantage of this window of opportunity. Once you have taught your baby how to fall asleep on her own at night, you can use the same techniques to improve naps.

- Look forward to some rest. Most babies who can fall asleep by themselves will start to sleep all the way through the night.

THE OVERWHELMING MAJORITY OF BABIES WHO CAN FALL ASLEEP ON THEIR OWN AT BEDTIME AND WHO ARE NOT FED IN THE MIDDLE OF THE NIGHT START TO SLEEP THROUGH UNTIL MORNING. interventions don't seriously hamper your own sleep, you can take a wait-and-see approach. Your baby may start to soothe herself back to sleep without crying when she's a little older—possibly a few weeks or a few months. Don't let anyone make you feel guilty for going to your baby at night if you've followed all the sleep training advice here and are using the N.A.P.S. plan. It may be small comfort when you're in the thick of this rough time, but what's most important is that you have a well-rested baby.

Naps: Falling Asleep, Staying Asleep

✳ Once your baby can fall asleep on her own at night, you can teach her the same skill at nap time. Self-soothing skills are basically the same for naps as for nights. A very brief nap-time routine, perhaps a book or a lullaby, is helpful. Keep it as short as possible. Then go ahead and start the self-soothing method of your choice. If your baby has learned how to fall asleep at night, she knows the drill and will probably fall asleep at nap time with much less crying, maybe without any protesting at all. That's good, because you'll definitely need to limit crying at nap times to about fifteen minutes. After that, the next 90-minute alertness phase will have started, and you'll have to try again at the next nap.

If your baby is on the N.A.P.S. plan but still takes very short naps during the day, you can also use self-soothing techniques to extend daytime sleep. Sometimes the baby needs to learn how to get over a

Andy's Story: *The Night Wakings Started to Get Worse*

"My wife and I had a friend who used the N.A.P.S. plan and recommended it to us enthusiastically. Our friend's baby had been on the program since he was a few weeks old, and he eventually learned to sleep through the night with just a few minutes of crying. This was very appealing to my wife and me. We didn't want to co-sleep, but we also didn't want to let our baby cry it out for a long time.

"When Joey was a newborn, the N.A.P.S. plan worked smoothly. Then at six months it came time to teach Joey how to fall asleep on his own and to sleep through the night. I was looking forward to this because I'm the one on night duty in our house. Luckily, Joey went down for the night after whimpering for maybe five minutes. My wife and I were proud of Joey and we congratulated ourselves on being such good parents. I sat back and waited for the nights to get better.

"They didn't. The night wakings started to get worse. He would wake up three or four times a night, and it was taking longer and longer to get him back in his crib each time. We both hated the idea of leaving a little baby to cry in the middle of the night, but something had to give. The next Friday night, Joey woke up in the late evening, but I didn't go in to him. I checked on him a few times, but that seemed to make him angrier, so I stopped. After fifteen minutes, he was still crying hard. I thought he needed more of a chance to calm himself down, so I watched television with the sound turned down low and waited. It was disturbing to hear him wail, but he did start to quiet down after about twenty minutes. Then came the frustrating part: He seemed to fall asleep, and then he woke up crying again five minutes later. He did this off and on for almost an hour. Eventually he went to sleep for good. The next night, he woke up and cried for ten minutes, period. The night after that, he slept straight through.

"When we talked to Polly about the difficulty Joey had, she reassured us. Some children have a harder time with sleep independence than others, and Joey probably got caught in a cycle of becoming agitated from his own crying. This was one of those parenting situations where there is no clear right or wrong thing to do. Some parents would have decided to go in and get him, and that would have been okay, but it was also okay for us to let him keep crying. I simply felt that all of us had been too miserable for too long and that it was worth enduring a really tough night for better sleep in the long term.

"Now Joey sleeps well as a general rule. I wouldn't want him to live that night over again, though."

20- or 30-minute nap hump. I can clearly remember when my daughter was still taking five short naps a day. I was ready for a change! First, I gave her opportunities for self-soothing at night. Once that was well established, I did the same at the onset of naps. She learned to put herself to sleep within a few days, and I gave her a week or two to solidify these skills. By this point, being awake in her crib was no longer distressing to her, so I then felt comfortable teaching her how to take longer naps. Here's how I did it: When my daughter awoke from her naps, I stopped going to her right away when she woke up. Instead, I gave her about fifteen minutes to soothe herself back to sleep. If she fell back asleep, great. If she sounded wide awake after fifteen minutes, I picked her up and assumed the alertness clock had started running again and put her back down 75 minutes later. Soon she was taking three naps a day: a morning and afternoon nap that each lasted two or three hours, and a quick evening nap.

Eight to Twelve Months

Just as you are getting the hang of parenthood, your baby up and does some growing on you! Although nap length and sleep amounts hold fairly steady at the end of the first year (on average, babies at this stage still need between thirteen and fourteen hours of sleep daily), you may have to handle a few curve balls caused by your baby's developments. Between eight and twelve months, most babies learn to creep, crawl, sit up, stand up, and possibly walk or talk. It's in their nature to respond with enthusiasm to these new abilities. You may see a spike in night wakings as the baby works out her newest trick or uses the bars of the crib to pull herself up. Try not to let these wakings throw you into a panic. When your baby wakes at night, respond as neutrally as you can, without giving the baby too much attention for demonstrating her new skills. Soon enough, these abilities won't be so new, and your baby will probably resume her former sleeping habits.

BETWEEN EIGHT AND TWELVE MONTHS, MOST BABIES LEARN TO CREEP, CRAWL, SIT UP, STAND UP, AND POSSIBLY WALK OR TALK. IT'S IN THEIR NATURE TO RESPOND WITH ENTHUSIASM TO THESE NEW ABILITIES.

Nap Maps for Ten-Month-Old Babies

As before, keep in mind that these "maps" represent sample days; they're not schedules that your baby must adhere to. Try to let your baby's sleep schedule take shape on its own.

MIA'S NAPS

At ten months, Mia has just now dropped her evening nap and developed a three-hour wakeful period between naps. Though some babies drop their nighttime nap sooner, Mia's timeline is perfectly normal and just right for her. (For Mia's naps at seven months of age, see page 95.)

Wake-up
7:00 AM

Morning nap
10:00 AM–11:30 AM

Afternoon nap
2:30 PM–3:30 PM

Bedtime
8:00 PM

JACK'S NAPS

Jack's schedule is similar to what it was at seven months (see page 95), though his naps have shifted a bit. His perceptive parents have realized that Jack actually prefers going to bed earlier now than he did a few months ago—a development that is unusual but perfectly normal—and they are happy to comply with his wishes.

Wake-up
6:00 AM

First nap
9:00 AM–10:30 AM

Second nap
1:30 PM–3:30 PM

Bedtime
6:30 PM

ISAAC'S NAPS

Isaac's schedule is the same now as it was when he was seven months old (see page 95): He remains awake for longer in the morning, and his wakeful periods between naps each last three hours.

Wake-up
6:30 AM

First nap
9:30 AM–11:00 AM

Second nap
2:00 PM–3:30 PM

Bedtime
8:00 PM

SLEEPING THROUGH THE NIGHT—AGAIN

✻ People talk about "sleeping through the night" as if it's a onetime accomplishment, but in reality your child will wake up at night plenty during the next several years: for developmental reasons; because of illness, teething, or bad dreams; or while traveling. If these wakings become habitual long after their causes have faded, you will need to reteach your child how to soothe herself.

If your baby has not yet learned how to fall asleep on her own, follow the instructions starting on page 94. Some babies are not ready to learn self-soothing until late in the first year, and you may sense when an optimum time approaches. Just know that older babies may protest more vociferously. They're cleverer now about how to get responses out

THE N.A.P.S. PLAN AT A GLANCE

Eight to Twelve Months

- Most babies at this age need somewhere between thirteen and fourteen hours of sleep daily. Your baby's needs may be somewhat lesser or greater.

- Continue to use the N.A.P.S. program. If your baby has not yet dropped her evening nap or developed longer wakeful periods throughout the day, she will probably do so soon.

- Don't pressure your baby to give up her morning nap. It may shorten, but most infants need a morning nap until they are twelve to eighteen months old.

- Be prepared for some rough spots at night during this age, especially when your infant develops new skills.

of you, and they may feel entitled to have you rock or soothe them all the way to sleep. But don't panic. It's never too late to teach your baby good sleep habits.

One Year and Beyond

After the first year of life, the 90-minute cycle tends to loosen its grip on sleepy behavior, but it's not as if it stops the minute your child blows out (or eats) the candle on his birthday cake. You will have to use your observations and instincts as your child grows out of a strict adherence to the cycle. Some hang on to it for a few months after their first birthday. A few parents can spot a three-hour pattern of alertness even when their toddlers are two or three. However, most children at this age start to develop schedules based on clock time, not 90-minute cycles. Perhaps you will continue to see a sleep rhythm, but it and your child will gradually grow more flexible. Getting your child into the crib or bed at the very first sign of fatigue may be less necessary as the months go by, although you should still honor your child's sleepiness. Sometimes a child seems to drop the 90-minute cycle, only to revert to it when ill or stressed. Some parents have noticed that toddlers who wake up sick at night are ready for sleep again 90 minutes later.

No matter how or when the 90-minute rhythm begins to phase out, sleep remains a deep biological need for your child. The average daily sleep need for one-year-olds is about thirteen hours. If you have followed the N.A.P.S. plan in the first year (even if you started in the tenth or eleventh month), you have helped your baby develop good sleep habits that will extend themselves into the toddler years, school years, and beyond.

Your child has the ability to sleep when she is sleepy—and to remain asleep as long as necessary. She knows what it's like to feel well rested; she may seek out sleep opportunities and even point to her crib or say "nighty-night" when she is tired. However, your toddler is also developing a new sense of her own power. It's normal for her to test the bedtime or nap rules now and then, and it remains your job to make sure she gets appropriate naps and has an early bedtime. But if your child understands how to interpret her own sleepiness and knows what to do about it, those bedtime battles are much less likely to escalate into the full-blown toddler sleep wars that are so common these days.

Be on the lookout for some nap-time changes as your baby grows into a toddler. Sometime between the first birthday and eighteen months of age, the morning nap drops out. Losing this nap can be rough for children and their parents; for a few days or even weeks, it may seem as if two naps are too much and one nap isn't quite sufficient. Give your toddler's brain adequate time to sort out this adjustment, and expect some cranky days and bumpy evenings until your child has fully made the transition.

Contrary to popular opinion, the afternoon nap should stick around for several years. You'll probably encounter a few people who think that a child's need for daytime sleep is a sign of inferiority or low intelligence, but nothing could be further from the truth. I wish I had a dollar for every time a parent of a toddler bragged to me that their three- or four-year-old has "outgrown" her nap or is "too smart" for it. Yes, some toddlers can stay awake during nap time, but when they do, their behavior often changes dramatically. They lose control of their impulses and temper, they become clumsy, they become intractable, they lose their ability to focus, they are quick to tears—sound familiar? In other words, the usual signs of sleepiness are still present. Be aware that simply being

NAP MAPS FOR EIGHTEEN-MONTH-OLD BABIES

These sample maps provide examples of how your child's sleep schedule might arrange itself by the eighteenth month of life. They are only examples, not schedules that your baby must follow.

MIA'S NAPS

Mia took a long time to drop her evening nap (see page 109), but she is the first of our nap map babies to stop napping in the morning. Her afternoon nap has moved up by several hours. Note that her wakefulness no longer occurs in 90-minute increments.

Wake-up
7:30 AM

Afternoon nap
Noon–3:00 PM

Bedtime
7:30 PM

JACK'S NAPS

Jack continues to have two naps, but his naps are shorter and his wakeful periods no longer come in increments of 90 minutes. His parents have therefore put him on a clock schedule, which suits Jack just fine. His bedtime, now 7:00 PM, is slightly later than it was at ten months of age (see page 109).

Wake-up
6:00 AM

First nap
9:00 AM–10:00 AM

Second nap
2:00 PM–3:00 PM

Bedtime
7:00 PM

ISAAC'S NAPS

Isaac maintains the schedule he's been on for several months now (see pages 95 and 109) and he continues to thrive on it.

Wake-up
6:30 AM

First nap
9:30 AM–11:00 AM

Second nap
2:00 PM–3:30 PM

Bedtime
8:00 PM

able to force wakefulness during nap-time hours is not a true indicator that your toddler no longer needs a nap. You must go by other clues!

Also take care when deciding which special events are worth skipping a nap for. The detrimental effects of a skipped nap are farther reaching than you may realize. A missed nap can disrupt your child's body clocks for a period that lasts longer than 24 hours. Know that there will be consequences of a missed nap for (1) the remainder of that day, (2) the sleep that follows that night, and (3) the ability to nap the next day.

 THE DETRIMENTAL EFFECTS OF A SKIPPED NAP ARE FARTHER REACHING THAN YOU MAY REALIZE. A MISSED NAP CAN DISRUPT YOUR CHILD'S BODY CLOCKS FOR A PERIOD THAT LASTS LONGER THAN 24 HOURS.

Please don't push your child to give up her nap early.

In some cases, toddlers around two and a half to three years of age suddenly give up their afternoon naps—but they also extend nighttime sleep by the amount of sleep they used to get at nap time. This shift of sleep from day to night is healthy and normal, as long as total sleep time during 24 hours stays the same and as long as you keep the child's schedule consistent from day to day. Just don't try to force a toddler to make the shift, and be sure to allow enough time at night for the new and longer sleep period. Toddlers who make this change may seem to do it "on their own," but in my opinion this is generally a response to the parents not providing a consistent nap time. Remember that in most mammals and in many cultures, the pull for a rest in the early afternoon is very strong and probably genetic. Make sure that giving up a nap is what's best for your toddler, not just for you.

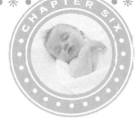

Personalize the Plan
Solving Common Sleep Problems

A baby's brain is like a delicately calibrated musical instrument, designed to beat out rhythmic patterns of sleep and alertness. These patterns are highly predictable, which is why the N.A.P.S. plan works quickly to improve sleep.

But each baby has a unique way of adapting to these cycles and to the conditions of the household. To help you fine-tune the N.A.P.S. plan according to your baby's needs, I've listed the most common sleep problems I see in babies, along with explanations and solutions. In some cases, the solution is very strict adherence to the plan. Sometimes a problem can be addressed by borrowing from other elements of sleep research. With a few quick lessons in how babies regulate their body heat or how their 24-hour circadian rhythms emerge, for example, you'll be more prepared to handle the puzzling sleep habits that may arise.

My Baby Cries Unless I Hold Him

Sleepiness can manifest itself in sneaky ways. One, described on pages 48 and 49, is "mystery fussiness," which is crying and grumbling that can't be traced to an obvious cause such as hunger or sickness. In newborns, this "fussiness" tends to take the form of out-and-out wailing. In babies who are three months and older, the baby may not actually cry or show tears; instead, the baby fusses and grumbles until he is picked up and held. Once he's in his parent's arms, he quiets—until he is put back down, when the fussing resumes.

This fussiness and desire to be held are two common signs of sleepiness, although they can be difficult for parents to interpret. After all, parents may think to themselves, how sleepy can the baby be if he stops whining when he's held? Parents often say to me, "My baby isn't tired, but he needs to be held all the time." Such a baby is, in fact, underslept. On some

PARENTS OFTEN SAY TO ME, "MY BABY ISN'T TIRED, BUT HE NEEDS TO BE HELD ALL THE TIME." SUCH A BABY IS, IN FACT, UNDERSLEPT.

level, he "knows" that he needs to sleep and, in a way, he also "knows" that he needs his parents to help him do so. This is why he fusses until a parent picks him up and why he's quiet once he's held. He's thinking, "Oh good, Dad's picked me up. He's going to help me get to sleep now."

One danger here is that parents will mistakenly attribute this behavior to a clingy or needy temperament, which may cause them to put a negative label on the child at a very early age. But when a supposedly clingy or high-need baby is given more sleep, parents are often surprised to find that the child's personality has completely changed! The baby is often much happier and starts to enjoy reasonable amounts of independent playtime. Even babies who are born with truly difficult personalities—the kind who are born screaming and never seem to take much of a break thereafter—will be calmer if their parents can help them get more time asleep.

My Baby Wakes Up Crying

Sleep-deprived children may wake up crying in the morning or at the end of their naps. If your baby regularly wakes up crying, check his total sleep time across the day and night, refer to the sleep chart on page 10, and then ask yourself whether he is adequately rested. Crying may be his way of saying, "I wish I could get back to sleep, but I can't do it on my own." If appropriate, encourage more sleep. Use the N.A.P.S. plan to help him sleep during the day, and consider moving his bedtime earlier in the evening to extend total night sleep. Some families I've worked with have set aside a few days to try to achieve this sleep extension.

However, waking up slowly (as opposed to waking up crying) does not *always* indicate insufficient sleep. Babies (as well as adults) differ in how long it takes them to become fully alert upon awakening. My seven-year-old son wakes up most mornings at exactly 6:40 AM, bright and cheerful. My daughter, who is now nine, is very different. Although she usually has a cheerful disposition at just about any other time of day, she can be grouchy when she first wakes up. Until the cobwebs clear, she's really not "herself."

Sleep researchers have a term for this kind of slow, grumpy wake-up. It's called sleep inertia. It's a cloudy, fuzzy state that usually fades after a few minutes, although some people need up to half an hour before they feel totally alert. This phenomenon is so common that sleep researchers often need to account for the effects of sleep inertia when they perform cognitive-performance studies on humans.

My Baby Wakes Up Too Early in the Morning

You may have noticed that some of your friends and relatives are early-rising larks, whereas others are night owls. No matter what the old wives' tales say, these preferences are genetic and not caused by personality traits such as industriousness, sociability, or laziness. Attempts to change or switch these preferences invariably fail.

Babies and children have a strong tendency to be larks—at least until the adolescent years, when they may exhibit a night-owl tendency. From a biological point of view, early awakening (that is, with the dawn, or even the predawn light) is healthy for young children. I realize this can be hard on parents, and believe me, I've been there with my own kids. But a young child's brain is designed to signal an early rising, perhaps to help adapt him to the 24-hour cycle of lightness and darkness of our planet. That's why so many babies wake up with the sun, full of energy, and grow sleepy at dusk.

There is a wide range of normal wake-up times, from 5:00 AM to 9:00 AM. How can you tell if your baby's early wake-up is healthy? His mood as the day goes on is a good indicator. A baby who is generally happy, able to focus and pay attention, is probably telling you that he's well rested and awakening naturally. There is little you can do to change a biologically driven early rising. I know of families so desperate to postpone their child's early waking that they completely covered the windows in the nursery. I don't recommend this as a rule. It's much bet-

> **IT'S MUCH BETTER TO GO WITH A BABY'S NATURAL EBB AND FLOW OF ALERTNESS AND SLEEPINESS THAN TO FIGHT IT OR TRICK IT WITH MISINFORMATION.**

ter to go with a baby's natural ebb and flow of alertness and sleepiness than to fight it or trick it with misinformation. Hang in there, keep the coffee pot within easy reach, and remember that your baby won't be in this stage forever. Most children start to sleep in later by the school years (which is just when you need them to wake up early to catch the bus!). A child who is often cranky throughout the day, however, may be awakening too early because he is not getting adequate sleep at other times during the day. If you suspect that your baby isn't well rested, *don't* attempt to delay awakening by moving the bedtime later. This rarely works, and often it produces an even earlier wake-up time. Here are a few strategies for extending morning sleep that are more likely to work:

Put the baby to bed earlier in the evening. It sounds crazy, but earlier bedtimes often lead to later wake-up times. To move your baby's bedtime up, start by putting the baby to bed fifteen minutes earlier than usual. If you are following the N.A.P.S. plan, you may need to wake your baby from his afternoon or evening nap fifteen minutes earlier to accomplish the earlier bedtime. This goes against my usual advice of allowing a baby to wake up naturally, but you will need to do this for only a few days. Push the bedtime up a little more each night until you see signs that the baby is fully rested upon awakening. When you reach this point, you may find that the baby's total sleep time is extended by 90 minutes, which is the time it takes to complete one sleep cycle.

Make sure the baby is napping enough during the day. This is another method that sounds illogical but works like a charm. Babies who don't get all their naps may wake up too early, sometimes well before dawn. Follow the N.A.P.S. plan and watch your baby's sleepy signals to make sure he's getting adequate daytime sleep.

Be wary of conditioning an early wake-up time with feedings. Regular 5:00 AM feedings can condition the body's hunger signals, contributing to an artificially early waking and perhaps cementing it, even if the child hasn't met his full sleep need. Use your good judgment about whether a feeding is truly necessary and not just your attempt to get a few more winks. Please don't interpret this to mean that it's wrong or bad to feed your baby in the early morning hours. Just consider that your short-term solution today may lead to a longer-term problem for the next few weeks, as your baby becomes accustomed to breakfast at five in the morning.

Make sure the baby's not cold. One study has shown that adults with cold toes have a harder time falling asleep at night, and there are other signs that body temperature affects sleep. We all regulate our body temperature poorly in REM sleep, and babies, because of their surface-to-volume ratio, lose heat more rapidly than big people do. This heat loss can cause them to wake up early, especially at the end of a REM cycle. Make sure your child's room is comfortably cool but not cold or drafty; in cooler weather, a blanket "footie" sleeper might keep the baby from jolting out of sleep too early.

In special circumstances only, try room-darkening shades. It's normal and healthy for babies to wake when the sun rises, so I'm usually reluctant to trick a child's circadian clock with room-darkening shades. Even if you do not get home until late in the evening, try to maintain an early bedtime for your child.

Try to use dark shades only if there are significant special circumstances—say, the baby shares a room with Grandma, who needs to sleep late for medical reasons. If you live in a northern latitude where the nights are sometimes short and sunrise occurs before 5:00 AM, your baby may not get adequate sleep unless the room is artificially darkened (or unless he goes to bed at 6:00 PM at night). And when you're following the N.A.P.S. plan and putting your baby to bed early at night but still feel that the baby is sleep deprived, blackout shades may be your only fallback. Not all babies respond to these shades, however.

My Baby Won't Respond to "Crying It Out" Methods

I believe it's important for your baby to learn how to soothe himself and fall asleep without your presence. Teaching your baby this skill usually involves waiting until an appropriate age, setting up a bedtime routine, and then allowing your drowsy-but-still-awake baby to fall asleep by himself. Because your baby may protest at first, this method is often called "crying it out" or "controlled crying" (it's also called "Ferberizing," after Dr. Richard Ferber, the most famous advocate of controlled crying). A detailed approach to the method can be found on pages 98 to 100.

Some experts talk about self-soothing methods as if they will always work for every baby, but some circumstances practically guarantee failure. Pages 97 to 98 have already described some of these obstacles, but some parents find the self-soothing so difficult and emotionally charged that it's worth taking another look at how to handle some of the problems that may come up during this process.

Trying to teach self-soothing when the baby is sick or when the family is going through a major change is never a good idea. Parental inconsistency is also a major culprit. The sleep-training process requires that you develop a plan and stick to it, even though you may feel discomfort as your baby protests this change of routine. Don't try to sneak in a snuggle halfway through the process or rock him to sleep "just this once." When you are inconsistent, you're only teaching your child that crying

THE SLEEP-TRAINING PROCESS REQUIRES THAT YOU DEVELOP A PLAN AND STICK TO IT, EVEN THOUGH YOU MAY FEEL DISCOMFORT AS YOUR BABY PROTESTS THIS CHANGE OF ROUTINE.

for a long time could be worth the effort because you just might come to him. And if the baby is in a room that is too cold, too hot, too noisy, or too bright, the baby will obviously have trouble going to sleep. But even parents who study the popular sleep manuals and follow all of the instructions to the letter can run into obstacles. *That's because many of the most popular self-soothing methods do not take a baby's sleep rhythms into account.* Ignoring sleep rhythms is a sure way to stack the odds of success against you.

One common myth is that babies should achieve sleep independence at three months of age or even earlier. This is too young for most babies to learn how to fall asleep on their own. At three months, it may be too hard for a baby to focus on his body's signals that it is time to sleep. But by around six months, a baby's nervous system is more mature, and he's better able to tune out and wind down.

Even if your baby has reached an appropriate age, self-soothing is unlikely to work if the baby is put down at the wrong time. Remember that the 90-minute clock dictates when your baby is alert and when he is most receptive to falling asleep. If you put your baby down when he is in the highly alert phase of the cycle, he will not be ready to sleep—and he'll probably cry with frustration at being left alone when he is fully awake. But if you follow his cycles, you will know when the baby is maximally sleepy and the chances of success are highest.

Another little-known fact is that self-soothing is unlikely to work if the baby is overtired. I work with many parents who say things like, "I tried controlled crying and the baby screamed miserably for hours every evening before I finally gave up." These parents feel like failures, even though they are careful to follow the self-soothing instructions, remaining steady and consistent through the process. As I inquire about the baby's sleep habits, it soon becomes clear that the baby isn't getting enough sleep, particularly during the day. These sleep-deprived babies are usually irritable and, as a consequence, they are more in need of cuddling than other infants. Putting these children into a crib on their own and expecting them to go to sleep is a recipe for trouble. Although it seems logical that a sleep-deprived child should be able to crash quickly, in fact, the opposite is true. Sleep deprivation produces a chronic state of unrest in the baby's brain and can make falling asleep much more difficult. In my opinion, it's a bad idea to take an overtired baby and then put him in a cry-it-out situation. The process will probably backfire, with the baby growing more and more upset the longer he is left alone.

If your goal is to pursue self-soothing and your child is overtired, first devote a few days to helping your child get adequate sleep, especially during the day. This is your primary goal and should be established first before moving on to the next step. You can accomplish this by following the N.A.P.S. plan, and for a few days do whatever it takes to help your child get daytime sleep, whether it's holding him in your arms as he sleeps, putting him in a sling, mechanical swing, or driving him around in the car. Then, once he's better rested, you can teach him how to sleep independently.

Finally, there appears to be a subgroup of normal, healthy children who are temperamentally unsuited for self-soothing methods that involve crying. Babies who are very social or persistent can be capable of protesting your absence for brutally long periods of time. Instead of gradually quieting down after some initial crying, these children ratchet up their cries as their distress starts to feed on itself. When this happens, you may make the determination that your child is too upset to console

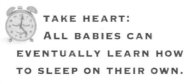

TAKE HEART: ALL BABIES CAN EVENTUALLY LEARN HOW TO SLEEP ON THEIR OWN.

himself. Use your judgment here, and be sure you aren't simply projecting your own emotions onto your child. At this point, you may decide to use a different self-soothing technique, such as facing. Fading takes much longer to work but involves a much more gradual reduction of your presence. Or you can call off the self-soothing process for now and wait until the baby is older, when he may be more accepting of change and independence. And take heart: All babies can eventually learn how to sleep on their own.

My Baby Can't Stay Up Late

If you've noticed that your baby is sleepy early in the evening, good for you. You've picked up on a common (and healthy) infant sleep pattern, which shows that you're attuned to your baby's sleep signals. Now you may need to adjust your expectations about what constitutes an appropriate bedtime. Although newborns may not begin night sleep until 10:00 or 11:00 PM, babies older than three months usually need an earlier bedtime—usually somewhere between 6:00 and 8:00 in the evening. Some parents are shocked to find that their child is able to fall asleep early in the evening and wonder if there's something wrong with the baby. Nothing is wrong. I think it's great when parents let their sleepy baby go down at 6:00 PM and maximize his nighttime rest.

You may know other babies who stay up very late, but young children who are natural night owls are rare. In most cases, babies who are awake after prime time have been conditioned by their parents or have inadvertently gotten a second wind from having missed the sleepy phase of the 90-minute cycle. This can sometimes happen when parents work outside the home and want to spend quality time with their children before bed. As a working mother myself, I understand this desire—but I nevertheless discourage parents from manipulating their babies' natural sleep rhythms. Doing so may result in sleep loss that could have detrimental long-term consequences. Instead, let your child sleep according to his developing circadian rhythms. For most children, this means going to bed at dusk (or earlier, especially in the summer, when daylight can linger well after the evening news) and waking in the morning light. Those early mornings can be tough on parents accustomed to keeping late hours, but look at them this way: They create an opportunity to spend time with your child when he is refreshed and playful, instead of grumpy or hyper from being kept up too late.

My Baby Gets a Second Wind Before Bedtime

If your baby experiences a surge of energy in the evening hours, don't chalk it up to bedtime resistance or bad luck—the real reason may be bad timing. If you miss the opportunity at the end of the alertness cycle to put your baby to bed, he will indeed develop a second wind, and you'll have a charged-up baby on your hands for another full wakeful cycle. Try moving the bedtime routine earlier in the evening, so you are ready to help your baby sleep or put him down in his crib at the end of the alertness cycle. You may find that the baby goes to sleep with less fussing. As a bonus, he may wake up later in the morning as well.

My Baby Takes Short Naps

Short naps of less than an hour can be frustrating for parents, but they are normal under some circumstances. For example, babies who are three months or older may have evening naps that often last for just thirty minutes. Short naps are also standard for many newborn babies, although most will take at least one longer nap sometime during the day. If your new baby catnaps but you don't have any other major concerns about his sleep, don't worry—but be aware of a few things.

First, new babies devote a high percentage of their sleep time to the REM stage, which is highly active and can resemble a wakeful state. They also spend a lot of time in a state that's not really sleep but isn't really wakefulness either. If you hear your baby stirring or even "talking" to you, try to wait a few minutes before picking him up. Despite appearances to the contrary, he may be sleeping. If not, he may be able to drift back into sleep by himself.

Second, use the N.A.P.S. plan to ensure that your catnapping baby gets enough total daytime sleep (see the sleep chart on page 10). This will result in several naps daily, and at this early age, that's fine. Don't cut back on his naps in an attempt to increase their length. By following his natural rhythms, your baby may learn to stretch out his sleep periods.

DON'T CUT BACK ON HIS NAPS IN AN ATTEMPT TO INCREASE THEIR LENGTH. BY FOLLOWING HIS NATURAL RHYTHMS, YOUR BABY MAY LEARN TO STRETCH OUT HIS SLEEP PERIODS.

Finally, you can always try rocking or soothing your newborn back to sleep when he wakes up from a short nap. This is more likely to work if he wakes up crying (a possible indication of sleep deprivation) than if he wakes up happy and ready to play.

If your baby is six months or older and still takes very short naps, you can use self-soothing techniques to extend nap length. For more information about self-soothing techniques and short naps, see pages 105 to 108.

Amy's Story: *My Baby Took 45-Minute Naps*

"When my daughter Hayley was a newborn, I used the N.A.P.S. plan to help her sleep. It was a good thing to follow because Hayley didn't have clearly distinct sleepy signs. When I started the program and she fell asleep, I'd ask myself, 'Now what did she sound like just before sleeping?' This helped me identify the difference between the cry that meant she was bored and the cry that meant she was sleepy.

"But there was another problem: Hayley took 45-minute naps. Even when I gave her six naps a day, she didn't get as much sleep as the charts said was necessary. Polly reminded me babies' sleep needs can vary. That made me feel better, and I relaxed a little.

"Now, I think that Hayley wanted to sleep for longer periods in the early months; she just didn't know how to do it. I used to go in to her when she woke up after 45 minutes and assume her nap was over. Then I decided to try soothing her back to sleep after the 45-minute mark. I would rock, cuddle, nurse—whatever it took. I found out that she would go back down for another 45 minutes or longer. And now Hayley does get the recommended amount of sleep for babies her age."

Occasionally I encounter parents whose babies catnap *and* whose feeding schedules take the form of very frequent sips rather than longer meals of milk or formula. Contrary to appearances, these "grazing" babies do not ingest more in a 24-hour period than babies fed at longer intervals and for longer periods of time. In fact, they may eat with less vigor than other babies do because they aren't allowed to build up an appetite. If this description fits your baby, encourage longer feeding sessions. If the baby is past the newborn stage, is developing well, and is gaining weight normally, ask your pediatrician's advice about gently extending the intervals between feedings—without, of course, ever letting your baby become desperately hungry. And ask yourself: Is my baby crying because he needs food, or could he be crying because he needs help going to sleep?

My Baby Won't Nap at All

A baby who doesn't take naps can be even more exhausting for parents than a baby who sleeps poorly at night. Fortunately, nature has designed babies to nap during the day. With some extra help from you, your baby can get the daytime sleep he needs.

Remember, the 90-minute clock promotes alertness, and at the end of the cycle, the alertness pressure is withdrawn. This is one of the reasons why it's so easy to deprive babies of their naps inadvertently. When a baby appears not to need naps, chances are that he's not being allowed to follow his natural sleep rhythms. If parents do not facilitate sleep at the end of the alertness cycle, they may miss the baby's window of opportunity for sleep. The parents may try to put him down later, at a time that disregards his internal rhythms, only to find it doesn't work.

The baby has skipped his nap and entered directly into the next alertness cycle, giving him the dreaded "second wind." When this happens continually, it may seem that the baby doesn't need to sleep—but believe me, he does. Some parents interpret this inability to sleep on cue as misbehavior. Others think that failure to nap is a sign of intelligence or an admirable perseverance in which the baby hates to sleep and fights naps with everything he's got. Really, though, what these babies need is the chance to sleep *when they are sleepy.* This opportunity occurs at the end of the alertness cycle, when it's easiest for the nervous system to switch to the brainwave patterns associated with sleeping.

Every now and then, parents tell me that they *enjoy* having their baby take irregular, unpredictable, and short naps because it gives them the flexibility to stay out for long periods during the day. A desire for more control over your day is understandable. It's really hard to adjust to scheduling life around a baby's demands. But the consequences of this practice could be serious. Fast forward to a year or so from now, when the baby starts to walk and is no longer content to hang out in the stroller, nodding off briefly now and then while you tend to business. Now you have a cranky and cantankerous toddler who won't sit in the stroller and whose chronic sleep deprivation is making every outing a disaster. At this point, you may wish you had dedicated more energy to establishing a decent nap program.

> **A DESIRE FOR MORE CONTROL OVER YOUR DAY IS UNDERSTANDABLE. IT'S REALLY HARD TO ADJUST TO SCHEDULING LIFE AROUND A BABY'S DEMANDS. BUT THE CONSEQUENCES OF THIS PRACTICE COULD BE SERIOUS.**

Worse, when babies aren't allowed to nap for a long period of time, their sleep/wake rhythms can flatten. In this state, sleep and alertness grow similar, creating a continuous in-between state in which the child is not asleep but also not fully focused and alert. Even the sleepy signals become less pronounced, so it's easy for a parent to conclude that the child "doesn't need" to sleep. That's why it's much easier to work with your baby on good sleep *now*.

To get your baby back on the nap track, make a commitment to staying home for a few days while you get the N.A.P.S. plan underway. Learn your baby's unique sleep signals (perhaps your baby has a hard-to-spot sleepy signal, such as minor inattentiveness or a vacant stare) and plan to devote some extra time to helping him block out the world's stimulation and drift off.

Once the naps are established, you may need to remain home for your baby's daytime sleep. You may have to do some creative rescheduling, but in the end you'll be thankful you did.

My Baby Needs Total Silence/Darkness to Sleep

B rand-new babies are famous for their ability to sleep in surprisingly loud and bright environments, and even older babies can zonk out during loud concerts and thunderstorms. But what about babies who awaken every time someone steps on a creaky floorboard, or turns on a hall light?

Sometimes a sensitive temperament is to blame. A few kids are simply unable to tolerate noise and light while sleeping. However, these babies are rare. Most cases of sensitive sleep are caused by too little sleep in the first place. Fatigue can lower the threshold of arousal and make a baby wake up too easily.

Before assuming that your baby is temperamentally sensitive, see if you can reverse the situation with good sleep management. Start the N.A.P.S. plan and stick to it. Your baby's need for complete darkness or silence may loosen up as he develops better sleep habits. If not, you may have a truly sensitive child who really does need a very dark, very quiet room. Try to accommodate this need to the extent possible.

My Baby Has Confused Day and Night

During the first eight weeks or so of life, it's normal for babies to have long periods of sleep in the day and shorter "naps" at night. (See page 65 for information about normal day/night confusion in new

 DURING THE FIRST EIGHT WEEKS OR SO OF LIFE, IT'S NORMAL FOR BABIES TO HAVE LONG PERIODS OF SLEEP IN THE DAY AND SHORTER "NAPS" AT NIGHT.

babies.) But some babies hang on to this confusion well into the third month. They may sleep for a block of six or eight hours during the day and wake up at night for frequent play periods. When this happens, you can carefully apply the 90-minute rhythm to ease your baby into a more appropriate pattern.

I suggest you begin by deciding when *you* want the baby to go to sleep for the night. That's what I did when my own kids were babies. For example, I wanted my babies to go to sleep for the night at my own bedtime so I could get my longest stretch of sleep at the same time they did. You'll work backward from that decision point, waking the baby from his nap 90 minutes before you want to go to bed. Let's say you want to sleep at 9:00 PM. When your baby starts taking one of those long daytime naps, make a note of the time. Then gently awaken the baby after three hours, which is the length of two 90-minute cycles. (I usually don't recommend that you awaken your baby from a nap, but this is a special circumstance.) Allow the baby to stay awake for a complete 90-minute cycle and then put him back down—and again, let him sleep for no longer than three hours and then keep him awake for 90 more minutes. By the end of this second long nap, it will probably be early in the evening. Put the baby down again, but wake him at 7:30 PM, no matter how short the nap has been. This way, he'll be tired again at 9:00 PM, and both you and he can go to sleep for the night.

If your baby doesn't have a long bout of sleep the first night, don't panic. It may take him a few nights to adjust. The good news is that your baby is capable of sleeping for several hours at a stretch. Soon enough, those hours will move to the night.

My Baby Sleeps Well, but Not When I Sleep

Your two- or three-month-old baby goes to sleep at 7:00 PM and doesn't have a night waking until 1:00 or 2:00 in the morning. What is there to complain about?

Plenty, if you don't go to bed until 9:00 or 10:00 at night. You get only a few good hours of slumber before receiving the call to duty. Again, I ordinarily do not suggest that parents manipulate their baby's sleep schedule, especially when the intent is merely to delay the time of the morning rising. But when a baby is still young and unable to sleep all the way through the night, there's some room to maneuver.

TO ENCOURAGE THE BABY'S LONGEST BOUT OF SLEEP TO LINE UP WITH YOUR OWN, USE THE 90-MINUTE CYCLE.

To encourage the baby's longest bout of sleep to line up with your own, use the 90-minute cycle. Ninety minutes before your chosen bedtime, wake the baby up. Ninety minutes later, he'll be ready to sleep again. With luck—and perhaps a few nights of practice with his new routine—he will sleep his accustomed six or seven hours.

When the baby's night sleep lengthens to eight or more hours straight, it's your cue to stop interrupting the baby's sleep in the early evening. Let him start bedtime according to his internal clock, and let him continue sleeping for as long as he wants.

My Baby Sleeps Only in the Car Seat/ Stroller/Swing/Sling

In the early weeks and months, you probably won't be able to avoid letting your baby fall asleep in the car seat or stroller at times. And I'm an advocate of using a sling or front pack with newborns, so long as they meet the weight requirements for the device. Slings and front packs give the baby a sense of security and can encourage natural, rhythmic sleep. They also allow you some freedom of movement. Try not to *depend* on the car seat, stroller, sling, or other device for the baby's sleep, however. It's an easy habit to develop but a hard one to live with in the long run. As the baby grows older, your shoulders and back will tire of wearing the baby for every single nap—and remember that babies quickly trade those portable infant car seats for heavier seats that can't be brought into the house for naps. And most—although not all—babies

AS THE BABY GROWS OLDER, YOUR SHOULDERS AND BACK WILL TIRE OF WEARING THE BABY FOR EVERY SINGLE NAP—AND REMEMBER THAT BABIES QUICKLY TRADE THOSE PORTABLE INFANT CAR SEATS FOR HEAVIER SEATS THAT CAN'T BE BROUGHT INTO THE HOUSE FOR NAPS. have shorter, shallower sleep in car seats and swings.

If it's too late and your baby is already addicted to an external device for sleep, examine the factors that make the device so appealing. Parents often wonder if it's the upright angle that the baby likes, but I suspect that babies love the warmth and coziness of front packs, slings, and even swings and car seats. Try using fitted flannel or knit sheets and a blanket sleeper to recreate this feeling in the crib or bassinet. If you have a newborn baby, try swaddling him tightly.

If those strategies don't work, you may need to wait until the baby is old enough to learn self-soothing (see pages 94 to 101 for more information). Until then, you might follow the example of one couple I know: They put the baby into the car seat, and put the car seat into the crib for several days. Eventually the baby developed a positive association with sleep and the crib.

My Baby Can't Stay Awake for 90 Minutes

Although many babies are born with a 90-minute cycle in place, some babies, especially babies born prematurely, have shorter cycles. Sickness or other disruptions may affect the clock as well. Go ahead and follow your baby's sleepy signals to determine nap times; don't ever try to force your baby to stay awake for 90 minutes. If your instincts tell you that your baby is sleeping too much or seems unusually lethargic, by all means check in with your doctor.

Babies of any age who have frequent sleep attacks accompanied by loss of muscle tone may be suffering from narcolepsy, a rare but serious sleep disorder. Another symptom of narcolepsy is falling asleep upon being excited. It's unusual to see symptoms of narcolepsy during infancy—most often the symptoms emerge during adolescence—but a few cases have been identified in babies. If your baby shows these symptoms, consult your doctor.

My Baby Won't Transfer from My Arms to the Crib

Young babies enter sleep directly into the REM sleep stage, which is lighter and more active than NREM sleep. Because it's easy to awaken from REM, a young baby who has just fallen asleep on your shoulder may wake up shortly after being put down in the bassinet. While in REM, a baby also has difficulty regulating his temperature. After getting warm and snuggly in your arms or while nursing, a baby may cool quickly when you put him down. The temperature change can also cause a premature waking. This can be frustrating for parents, but it helps to know that sleeping babies who don't transfer easily into a crib are perfectly normal.

A few techniques may help your baby make the transition from your arms into a crib. While soothing the baby, place a blanket between your body and the baby's, so it will grow warm from your body heat. Then, when you place the baby in the crib, leave the toasty blanket in with him. (Make sure that you are using a small light blanket, such as a receiving blanket, that is safe for babies.) Maintain as much body contact with the sleeping baby as you can as you ease him into the crib. Leave your hands on him for a few moments to make the transition less abrupt. A fitted knit or flannel sheet and a blanket sleeper may also help keep him warm; newborns will probably like to be swaddled. Another trick I used in the very early months was to nurse my daughter while I was lying down, having spread out the baby's blanket underneath her before we began. Once she fell asleep, I picked up the edges of the blanket, hammock style, and was able to put her into her bassinet gently without jostling her floppy neck or other tiny body parts and awakening her in the process. This method is particularly useful if your wrists are aching from holding the baby.

My Baby Wakes Up Frequently at Night

Until your baby is around six weeks old, expect frequent night wakings. These rounds of waking and sleeping may actually help the baby's brain calibrate the sleep mechanisms he'll use for the rest of his life.

After the first few months, some babies continue to wake up frequently, even when they are not ill. Parents often attribute these wakings to teething, gas pain, or emotional distress, but in my opinion these so-called causes are dubious.

There are three common patterns to frequent wakings: waking up every hour or two, waking up and eating voraciously, and waking up and falling asleep immediately after feeding has begun. In all cases, first make sure that the baby's sleeping environment is comfortable—not too cold and not too hot. Then you can try a few strategies that address your baby's specific pattern.

Waking Up Every Hour or Two. I've seen families in which the babies take just a few twenty-minute naps during the day, are up nearly every hour at night, and require nearly continuous holding and soothing. These are families for whom sleep deprivation has reached crisis proportions. The babies are unhappy, and the parents are zombies who are more than a little depressed and clearly unsafe to drive.

Because you may not have much control over nighttime sleep yet, focus on giving the baby better naps during the day. When he is better rested from good naps, his nights will improve. So follow the N.A.P.S. plan strictly, watching your baby like a hawk for signs of sleepiness. Even if you can't see any sleepy signals (and they may be hard to detect if he is crying a lot anyway), start the soothing process around five minutes before the 90-minute alertness cycle is over. Your baby may be harder to soothe than others, so consider yourself an exception and don't feel guilty if you have to rely on swings or constant use of a sling for a period of time, say a few days or a week. You can wean the baby from these external devices later. (Just don't depend on car rides if you're too tired to get behind the wheel.) Finally, take a look

> **YOUR BABY MAY BE HARDER TO SOOTHE THAN OTHERS, SO CONSIDER YOURSELF AN EXCEPTION AND DON'T FEEL GUILTY IF YOU HAVE TO RELY ON SWINGS OR CONSTANT USE OF A SLING FOR A PERIOD OF TIME, SAY A FEW DAYS OR A WEEK.**

at the advice on page 127 ("My Baby Takes Short Naps") if the catnaps persist and appear to leave your baby unrefreshed.

Waking Up Frequently—and Eating Voraciously. "My baby eats so much at night, he must be starving!" one mother said to me. This little boy was past the newborn period, in the 95th weight percentile, and clearly not suffering from weight-gain problems. I suggested that she consider another cause of the wakings: She had trained his digestive system to expect food by offering a bottle at each waking. He'd become dependent on the food to get back to sleep.

To reduce this dependence, you can cautiously use your instincts and good sense about offering comfort instead of food during night wakings. When the baby stops expecting constant snacks during the night, he may reduce the number of nighttime arousals. (Before following this advice, check with your pediatrician to be sure your baby is at an appropriate age and does not have a problem gaining weight.) For more information about night feedings and their connection to problematic wakings, see pages 84 to 88.

Waking Frequently but Falling Asleep Immediately After Feeding Has Begun. The baby wakes up; you offer a bottle or the breast, and within seconds the baby is asleep again. When this happens, you have a valuable set of clues. These clues point to the possibility that your baby isn't really hungry; he may just want some comfort to help him back into sleep. By feeding a baby who is six months or older frequently throughout the night, you may be creating a connection between food and sleep, or of needing an external source of comfort to fall asleep, and this perpetuates the night wakings. (Newborn babies, however, have a genuine need to eat often in the night.) By offering an alternative form of comfort, you can ease your baby off this habit, and the baby may start to sleep for longer periods on his own.

My Baby Used to Be a Good Sleeper, But Now He Wakes Up at Night

It can be crushing when a baby who was sleeping well suddenly starts to wake up again. You've had a taste of good sleep, and now you feel ripped off!

Unfortunately, there are almost always some blips in the sleep process—times when your baby wakes up even though he is not sick or hasn't been thrust out of sleep by an unusual event, such as a loud thunderstorm. These blips can occur during developmental milestones when the baby is learning to roll over, sit up, or stand up. He's excited and may want to share his happiness with you! Wakings may also occur during teething (although teething is overrated as a cause of serial wakings) or when a baby suffers from jet lag. Sometimes babies start waking up for reasons that no one fully understands.

Of course, if your baby is waking up because he is sick or in pain—you can probably tell by the cry, which tends to be much more insistent or higher pitched than usual—go to him and help him. If you have ruled out these causes and the baby is younger than six months, you may also need to attend to the baby. He's still very little and profoundly depen-dent on you. If he's already proven that he doesn't need to eat at night, try not to rely on food as a soothing method. Instead, comfort him with as little fuss as possible. In a few nights, he may resume his good sleeping habits. As a last resort, you can try letting the baby fuss for five or ten minutes before responding to him, especially if the cry sounds sleepy—he may settle down on his own. If that doesn't work, you may need to wait until he is old enough to learn self-soothing techniques.

If the baby is six months or older, you have a slightly different set of tools in your kit. Try giving the baby a few minutes to return to sleep before going in. Then respond as neutrally as possible. Try patting the baby without picking him up or talking to him in soothing tones. If the baby has pulled himself to a standing position and is unable to get down (it really happens), or if he has a foot caught between the crib slats, assist him and then try to leave the room I recommend doing this in as matter-of-fact a manner as possible. Try not to speak, don't smile, avoid making eye contact, and don't linger, because you don't want your baby to get the idea that it's time to play. If the baby is still waking up after a few nights, you may choose to teach him self-soothing techniques. If you have already gone through a self-soothing routine before, there's some good news: It should proceed more quickly this time.

My Baby Wants to Stay Awake Longer Than 90 Minutes

You may be right. By four months, many babies are ready to extend their evening wakefulness period from 90 minutes to three hours or even four and a half hours. Some will also have a three-hour period of alertness right after they wake up in the morning, especially if they are taking long naps. At around six months, yet another three-hour wakeful period may emerge between the morning and afternoon naps. Note, though, that the emergence of longer alertness periods happens on its own timeline. Your baby is not abnormal if he extends his wakefulness cycles earlier or later than the ages given here.

My Baby Doesn't Need as Much Sleep as You Say He Does

It's funny: Some babies don't read the sleep charts! Although most babies sleep a predictable number of hours in the day, some need more than the average and some need less. All babies, however, follow the 90-minute cycle in a developmentally appropriate way.

Before concluding that your baby needs less sleep than others do, make sure you are adhering to the N.A.P.S. plan, and that you are watching for and responding with alacrity to his signs of sleepiness. Don't expect the baby to conform to an adult's schedule, especially when it comes to daytime activities and bedtime. Do not cut off naps by taking the baby with you on too many errands and appointments, and try putting him to bed early to increase the number of hours he sleeps at night. You may be surprised at how much your baby can sleep when he is given the opportunity to follow his own body rhythms.

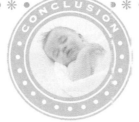
Get into the Rhythm

ountless parents have told me how easy it is to follow the N.A.P.S. plan. It's natural, however, to have your doubts and fears about the program: "How could my baby possibly go to sleep after 90 minutes of wakefulness? How can daytime naps improve nighttime sleep? How can I devote time to my baby's sleep when I'm so drained and exhausted?" If you are certain that the program could never work in your house, take a deep breath and think about this:

The first step is to feel positive about letting your baby sleep according to his inner rhythms. Remember that we all have natural cycles of rest and activity, and for good reason. The famous Ecclesiastes verse, "To everything there is a season/And a time for every purpose under heaven," reflects a truth known to the worlds great religious and philosophical systems: Not a single one of us is designed to go, go, go all the time. We all need time for active play, engaged learning, quiet day-dreaming, *and* restful slumber.

The second step is to get started! The N.A.P.S. plan may feel odd to you at first, but it quickly gets easier as you literally get into the rhythm. Even with the pressures and responsibilities of daily life, you will find it far easier in the long run to have a well-rested child than to ignore good sleep habits. You can do it; I *promise* you that you can do it and that it will improve your baby's—and your family's—sleep. Good luck, and sweet dreams.

Your Baby's
·S·L·E·E·P·
Journal

When you become aware of your baby's sleepy signals and sleep patterns, both you and your baby are well on the road to better, longer sleep. Keeping a log makes this task easier. In the first year of parenthood, you have a lot on your mind, like trying to remember which day of the week it is and whether your shoes match. (Tip: Don't worry too much about the shoes.) Even if you have a crackerjack memory in your normal life, you may find it hard to recall a day's and night's worth of your baby's sleep times if you don't write them down.

That's why I've provided a series of sleep logs for you on the following pages. They give you a designated place to jot down the times your baby has slept and the kind of behavior he's shown just before nodding off. Keep the log and a pencil where you are most likely to see them and use them, such as near the crib, co-sleeper, or wherever your baby sleeps.

One obvious benefit to using the sleep logs is that you will be able to spot emerging patterns more quickly. You can use this new awareness to guide your baby into sleep when he is most likely to go down easily and before he is in the crabby, hard-to-soothe state of being overtired. There are a few other advantages to the sleep logs. They can help you avoid common exaggerations like these: "My baby *never* sleeps" or "My baby cries *all* the time." Sleep logs can quickly correct your perceptions and help you feel better about your baby and your abilities as a parent. Also, spouses and babysitters may doubt that your baby really needs to sleep as much as you say he does. Sleep journals give you concrete proof that your baby really does follow a 90-minute sleep/wake cycle, or that, strange as it sounds to adults, your baby tends to pull on his ears (or perform some other odd behavior) when he's ready for sleep.

Because your baby's sleep patterns will evolve as the first year progresses, I've included logs for several distinct stages: the first two weeks, two weeks to three months, three months through five months, six months to eight months, and eight months to one year and beyond. *To use the logs, simply note the times that your baby sleeps: Write each of his wake times in the Waking Time column, and the start time of naps and bedtime in the Sleeping Time column—see right for a sample.* (I focus on nap times in this book, but I've left spaces for you to mark nighttime sleep and wakings if you choose.) You can use the additional lines provided to note your baby's sleepy signals, which may also change as your baby grows. When you are satisfied that you are tuned into your baby's sleep needs, you can put the journal away until you sense that his sleep patterns are changing and want to start keeping track again.

Keeping close track of your baby's sleep may feel odd at first—and in fact you will probably forget to note a few naps here and there. But I hope you will conclude that the minimal effort of maintaining a log for a few days at a time is worth the huge payoff of having a happy, well-rested child.

The First

Day Two	Waking Time	Sleeping Time
Midnight to 1:00 AM		
1:00 AM to 2:00 AM		
2:00 AM to 3:00 AM		
3:00 AM to 4:00 AM		
4:00 AM to 5:00 AM		
5:00 AM to 6:00 AM		
6:00 AM to 7:00 AM		
7:00 AM to 8:00 AM	7:30	
8:00 AM to 9:00 AM		9:00
9:00 AM to 10:00 AM	9:20	
10:00 AM to 11:00 AM		10:50
11:00 AM to Noon		
Noon to 1:00 PM		
1:00 PM to 2:00 PM	1:50	
2:00 PM to 3:00 PM		
3:00 PM to 4:00 PM		3:20
4:00 PM to 5:00 PM	4:00	
5:00 PM to 6:00 PM		5:30
6:00 PM to 7:00 PM	6:00	
7:00 PM to 8:00 PM		7:30
8:00 PM to 9:00 PM		
9:00 PM to 10:00 PM	9:30	
10:00 PM to 11:00 PM		11:00
11:00 PM to Midnight		

The First Two Weeks

SLEEP SIGNALS IN THE FIRST TWO WEEKS

Here, you can write down what your baby does or how he acts just prior to sleeping. In the first two weeks, many babies simply fall asleep on their own, or they may cry when they are tired.

_For more information about sleep signals and sleep patterns
in the first two weeks, see pages 62 to 68._

The First Two Weeks

AND NIGHTS IN THE
FIRST TWO WEEKS

Following is a week's worth of pages for you to track your baby's sleep during the first two weeks of life. It's fine if you don't feel the need to track your baby's sleep for seven whole days. During this period, you may see the 90-minute cycle emerging—or you may not. Just do your best to help the baby sleep, and try to get some rest yourself.

To use these logs, simply note the times that your baby sleeps: Write each of his wake times in the Waking Time column, and the start time of his naps and bedtime in the Sleeping Time column.

■ Day One	Waking Time	Sleeping Time
Midnight to 1:00 AM		
1:00 AM to 2:00 AM		
2:00 AM to 3:00 AM		
3:00 AM to 4:00 AM		
4:00 AM to 5:00 AM		
5:00 AM to 6:00 AM		
6:00 AM to 7:00 AM		
7:00 AM to 8:00 AM		
8:00 AM to 9:00 AM		
9:00 AM to 10:00 AM		
10:00 AM to 11:00 AM		
11:00 AM to Noon		
Noon to 1:00 PM		
1:00 PM to 2:00 PM		
2:00 PM to 3:00 PM		
3:00 PM to 4:00 PM		
4:00 PM to 5:00 PM		
5:00 PM to 6:00 PM		
6:00 PM to 7:00 PM		
7:00 PM to 8:00 PM		
8:00 PM to 9:00 PM		
9:00 PM to 10:00 PM		
10:00 PM to 11:00 PM		
11:00 PM to Midnight		

■ Day Two	Waking Time	Sleeping Time
Midnight to 1:00 AM		
1:00 AM to 2:00 AM		
2:00 AM to 3:00 AM		
3:00 AM to 4:00 AM		
4:00 AM to 5:00 AM		
5:00 AM to 6:00 AM		
6:00 AM to 7:00 AM		
7:00 AM to 8:00 AM		
8:00 AM to 9:00 AM		
9:00 AM to 10:00 AM		
10:00 AM to 11:00 AM		
11:00 AM to Noon		
Noon to 1:00 PM		
1:00 PM to 2:00 PM		
2:00 PM to 3:00 PM		
3:00 PM to 4:00 PM		
4:00 PM to 5:00 PM		
5:00 PM to 6:00 PM		
6:00 PM to 7:00 PM		
7:00 PM to 8:00 PM		
8:00 PM to 9:00 PM		
9:00 PM to 10:00 PM		
10:00 PM to 11:00 PM		
11:00 PM to Midnight		

■ Day Three	Waking Time	Sleeping Time
Midnight to 1:00 AM		
1:00 AM to 2:00 AM		
2:00 AM to 3:00 AM		
3:00 AM to 4:00 AM		
4:00 AM to 5:00 AM		
5:00 AM to 6:00 AM		
6:00 AM to 7:00 AM		
7:00 AM to 8:00 AM		
8:00 AM to 9:00 AM		
9:00 AM to 10:00 AM		
10:00 AM to 11:00 AM		
11:00 AM to Noon		
Noon to 1:00 PM		
1:00 PM to 2:00 PM		
2:00 PM to 3:00 PM		
3:00 PM to 4:00 PM		
4:00 PM to 5:00 PM		
5:00 PM to 6:00 PM		
6:00 PM to 7:00 PM		
7:00 PM to 8:00 PM		
8:00 PM to 9:00 PM		
9:00 PM to 10:00 PM		
10:00 PM to 11:00 PM		
11:00 PM to Midnight		

◼ **Day Four**	Waking Time	Sleeping Time	◼ **Day Five**	Waking Time	Sleeping Time
Midnight to 1:00 AM			Midnight to 1:00 AM		
1:00 AM to 2:00 AM			1:00 AM to 2:00 AM		
2:00 AM to 3:00 AM			2:00 AM to 3:00 AM		
3:00 AM to 4:00 AM			3:00 AM to 4:00 AM		
4:00 AM to 5:00 AM			4:00 AM to 5:00 AM		
5:00 AM to 6:00 AM			5:00 AM to 6:00 AM		
6:00 AM to 7:00 AM			6:00 AM to 7:00 AM		
7:00 AM to 8:00 AM			7:00 AM to 8:00 AM		
8:00 AM to 9:00 AM			8:00 AM to 9:00 AM		
9:00 AM to 10:00 AM			9:00 AM to 10:00 AM		
10:00 AM to 11:00 AM			10:00 AM to 11:00 AM		
11:00 AM to Noon			11:00 AM to Noon		
Noon to 1:00 PM			Noon to 1:00 PM		
1:00 PM to 2:00 PM			1:00 PM to 2:00 PM		
2:00 PM to 3:00 PM			2:00 PM to 3:00 PM		
3:00 PM to 4:00 PM			3:00 PM to 4:00 PM		
4:00 PM to 5:00 PM			4:00 PM to 5:00 PM		
5:00 PM to 6:00 PM			5:00 PM to 6:00 PM		
6:00 PM to 7:00 PM			6:00 PM to 7:00 PM		
7:00 PM to 8:00 PM			7:00 PM to 8:00 PM		
8:00 PM to 9:00 PM			8:00 PM to 9:00 PM		
9:00 PM to 10:00 PM			9:00 PM to 10:00 PM		
10:00 PM to 11:00 PM			10:00 PM to 11:00 PM		
11:00 PM to Midnight			11:00 PM to Midnight		

The First Two Weeks

■ Day Six	Waking Time	Sleeping Time
Midnight to 1:00 AM		
1:00 AM to 2:00 AM		
2:00 AM to 3:00 AM		
3:00 AM to 4:00 AM		
4:00 AM to 5:00 AM		
5:00 AM to 6:00 AM		
6:00 AM to 7:00 AM		
7:00 AM to 8:00 AM		
8:00 AM to 9:00 AM		
9:00 AM to 10:00 AM		
10:00 AM to 11:00 AM		
11:00 AM to Noon		
Noon to 1:00 PM		
1:00 PM to 2:00 PM		
2:00 PM to 3:00 PM		
3:00 PM to 4:00 PM		
4:00 PM to 5:00 PM		
5:00 PM to 6:00 PM		
6:00 PM to 7:00 PM		
7:00 PM to 8:00 PM		
8:00 PM to 9:00 PM		
9:00 PM to 10:00 PM		
10:00 PM to 11:00 PM		
11:00 PM to Midnight		

■ Day Seven	Waking Time	Sleeping Time
Midnight to 1:00 AM		
1:00 AM to 2:00 AM		
2:00 AM to 3:00 AM		
3:00 AM to 4:00 AM		
4:00 AM to 5:00 AM		
5:00 AM to 6:00 AM		
6:00 AM to 7:00 AM		
7:00 AM to 8:00 AM		
8:00 AM to 9:00 AM		
9:00 AM to 10:00 AM		
10:00 AM to 11:00 AM		
11:00 AM to Noon		
Noon to 1:00 PM		
1:00 PM to 2:00 PM		
2:00 PM to 3:00 PM		
3:00 PM to 4:00 PM		
4:00 PM to 5:00 PM		
5:00 PM to 6:00 PM		
6:00 PM to 7:00 PM		
7:00 PM to 8:00 PM		
8:00 PM to 9:00 PM		
9:00 PM to 10:00 PM		
10:00 PM to 11:00 PM		
11:00 PM to Midnight		

Two Weeks to Three Months

❋ ● ❋ ● ❋ ● ❋ ● ❋ ● ❋ ● ❋ ● ❋ ● ❋ ● ❋ ● ❋ ● ❋ ● ❋ ● ❋ ● ❋ ● ❋ ●

SLEEP SIGNALS FROM TWO WEEKS TO THREE MONTHS

Here you can write down what your baby does or how he acts just before sleeping. At this age, most babies cry when they are sleepy, but a few develop more subtle or unusual signs, such as pulling on their ears or staring into space.

For more information about sleep signals and sleep patterns
from two weeks to three months, see pages 69 to 79.

NOTE THE NAPS AND NIGHTS FROM TWO WEEKS TO THREE MONTHS

Here are a week's worth of pages for you to track your baby's sleep. It's fine if you don't feel the need to track your baby's sleep for seven whole days. In this period of your baby's life, you will likely see the emergence of the 90-minute cycle.

To use these logs, simply note the times that your baby sleeps: Write each of his wake times in the Waking Time column, and the start time of his naps and bedtime in the Sleeping Time column.

■ Day One	Waking Time	Sleeping Time
Midnight to 1:00 AM		
1:00 AM to 2:00 AM		
2:00 AM to 3:00 AM		
3:00 AM to 4:00 AM		
4:00 AM to 5:00 AM		
5:00 AM to 6:00 AM		
6:00 AM to 7:00 AM		
7:00 AM to 8:00 AM		
8:00 AM to 9:00 AM		
9:00 AM to 10:00 AM		
10:00 AM to 11:00 AM		
11:00 AM to Noon		
Noon to 1:00 PM		
1:00 PM to 2:00 PM		
2:00 PM to 3:00 PM		
3:00 PM to 4:00 PM		
4:00 PM to 5:00 PM		
5:00 PM to 6:00 PM		
6:00 PM to 7:00 PM		
7:00 PM to 8:00 PM		
8:00 PM to 9:00 PM		
9:00 PM to 10:00 PM		
10:00 PM to 11:00 PM		
11:00 PM to Midnight		

Two Weeks to Three Months

■ **Day Two**	Waking Time	Sleeping Time	■ **Day Three**	Waking Time	Sleeping Time
Midnight to 1:00 AM			Midnight to 1:00 AM		
1:00 AM to 2:00 AM			1:00 AM to 2:00 AM		
2:00 AM to 3:00 AM			2:00 AM to 3:00 AM		
3:00 AM to 4:00 AM			3:00 AM to 4:00 AM		
4:00 AM to 5:00 AM			4:00 AM to 5:00 AM		
5:00 AM to 6:00 AM			5:00 AM to 6:00 AM		
6:00 AM to 7:00 AM			6:00 AM to 7:00 AM		
7:00 AM to 8:00 AM			7:00 AM to 8:00 AM		
8:00 AM to 9:00 AM			8:00 AM to 9:00 AM		
9:00 AM to 10:00 AM			9:00 AM to 10:00 AM		
10:00 AM to 11:00 AM			10:00 AM to 11:00 AM		
11:00 AM to Noon			11:00 AM to Noon		
Noon to 1:00 PM			Noon to 1:00 PM		
1:00 PM to 2:00 PM			1:00 PM to 2:00 PM		
2:00 PM to 3:00 PM			2:00 PM to 3:00 PM		
3:00 PM to 4:00 PM			3:00 PM to 4:00 PM		
4:00 PM to 5:00 PM			4:00 PM to 5:00 PM		
5:00 PM to 6:00 PM			5:00 PM to 6:00 PM		
6:00 PM to 7:00 PM			6:00 PM to 7:00 PM		
7:00 PM to 8:00 PM			7:00 PM to 8:00 PM		
8:00 PM to 9:00 PM			8:00 PM to 9:00 PM		
9:00 PM to 10:00 PM			9:00 PM to 10:00 PM		
10:00 PM to 11:00 PM			10:00 PM to 11:00 PM		
11:00 PM to Midnight			11:00 PM to Midnight		

Two Weeks to Three Months

■ **Day Four**	Waking Time	Sleeping Time
Midnight to 1:00 AM		
1:00 AM to 2:00 AM		
2:00 AM to 3:00 AM		
3:00 AM to 4:00 AM		
4:00 AM to 5:00 AM		
5:00 AM to 6:00 AM		
6:00 AM to 7:00 AM		
7:00 AM to 8:00 AM		
8:00 AM to 9:00 AM		
9:00 AM to 10:00 AM		
10:00 AM to 11:00 AM		
11:00 AM to Noon		
Noon to 1:00 PM		
1:00 PM to 2:00 PM		
2:00 PM to 3:00 PM		
3:00 PM to 4:00 PM		
4:00 PM to 5:00 PM		
5:00 PM to 6:00 PM		
6:00 PM to 7:00 PM		
7:00 PM to 8:00 PM		
8:00 PM to 9:00 PM		
9:00 PM to 10:00 PM		
10:00 PM to 11:00 PM		
11:00 PM to Midnight		

■ **Day Five**	Waking Time	Sleeping Time
Midnight to 1:00 AM		
1:00 AM to 2:00 AM		
2:00 AM to 3:00 AM		
3:00 AM to 4:00 AM		
4:00 AM to 5:00 AM		
5:00 AM to 6:00 AM		
6:00 AM to 7:00 AM		
7:00 AM to 8:00 AM		
8:00 AM to 9:00 AM		
9:00 AM to 10:00 AM		
10:00 AM to 11:00 AM		
11:00 AM to Noon		
Noon to 1:00 PM		
1:00 PM to 2:00 PM		
2:00 PM to 3:00 PM		
3:00 PM to 4:00 PM		
4:00 PM to 5:00 PM		
5:00 PM to 6:00 PM		
6:00 PM to 7:00 PM		
7:00 PM to 8:00 PM		
8:00 PM to 9:00 PM		
9:00 PM to 10:00 PM		
10:00 PM to 11:00 PM		
11:00 PM to Midnight		

Two Weeks to Three Months

■ Day Six	Waking Time	Sleeping Time
Midnight to 1:00 AM		
1:00 AM to 2:00 AM		
2:00 AM to 3:00 AM		
3:00 AM to 4:00 AM		
4:00 AM to 5:00 AM		
5:00 AM to 6:00 AM		
6:00 AM to 7:00 AM		
7:00 AM to 8:00 AM		
8:00 AM to 9:00 AM		
9:00 AM to 10:00 AM		
10:00 AM to 11:00 AM		
11:00 AM to Noon		
Noon to 1:00 PM		
1:00 PM to 2:00 PM		
2:00 PM to 3:00 PM		
3:00 PM to 4:00 PM		
4:00 PM to 5:00 PM		
5:00 PM to 6:00 PM		
6:00 PM to 7:00 PM		
7:00 PM to 8:00 PM		
8:00 PM to 9:00 PM		
9:00 PM to 10:00 PM		
10:00 PM to 11:00 PM		
11:00 PM to Midnight		

■ Day Seven	Waking Time	Sleeping Time
Midnight to 1:00 AM		
1:00 AM to 2:00 AM		
2:00 AM to 3:00 AM		
3:00 AM to 4:00 AM		
4:00 AM to 5:00 AM		
5:00 AM to 6:00 AM		
6:00 AM to 7:00 AM		
7:00 AM to 8:00 AM		
8:00 AM to 9:00 AM		
9:00 AM to 10:00 AM		
10:00 AM to 11:00 AM		
11:00 AM to Noon		
Noon to 1:00 PM		
1:00 PM to 2:00 PM		
2:00 PM to 3:00 PM		
3:00 PM to 4:00 PM		
4:00 PM to 5:00 PM		
5:00 PM to 6:00 PM		
6:00 PM to 7:00 PM		
7:00 PM to 8:00 PM		
8:00 PM to 9:00 PM		
9:00 PM to 10:00 PM		
10:00 PM to 11:00 PM		
11:00 PM to Midnight		

Three Through Five Months

* ❋ * ❋ * ❋ * ❋ * ❋ * ❋ * ❋ * ❋ * ❋ * ❋ * ❋ * ❋ * ❋ *

SLEEP SIGNALS FROM THREE THROUGH FIVE MONTHS

Here you can write down what your baby does or how he acts just prior to sleeping. Your baby may now develop sleepy signals other than crying.

_____

_____

_____

_____

_____

_____

_____

_____

_____

_____

_____

_____

_____

_____

_____

_____

_____

_____

For more information about sleep signals and sleep patterns
from three through five months, see pages 80 to 92.

Here are a week's worth of pages for
you to track your baby's sleep. It's fine
if you don't feel the need to track it
for seven whole days. At around four
months, many babies will extend one
or more of their wakefulness periods
from 90 minutes to three hours or
four and a half hours. A longer period
of alertness often first appears in the
evening. Expect a few bumpy days as
your baby's brain sorts through this
change.

To use these logs, simply note
the times that your baby sleeps: Write
each of his wake times in the Waking
Time column, and the start time of his
naps and bedtime in the Sleeping Time
column.

■ Day One	Waking Time	Sleeping Time
Midnight to 1:00 AM		
1:00 AM to 2:00 AM		
2:00 AM to 3:00 AM		
3:00 AM to 4:00 AM		
4:00 AM to 5:00 AM		
5:00 AM to 6:00 AM		
6:00 AM to 7:00 AM		
7:00 AM to 8:00 AM		
8:00 AM to 9:00 AM		
9:00 AM to 10:00 AM		
10:00 AM to 11:00 AM		
11:00 AM to Noon		
Noon to 1:00 PM		
1:00 PM to 2:00 PM		
2:00 PM to 3:00 PM		
3:00 PM to 4:00 PM		
4:00 PM to 5:00 PM		
5:00 PM to 6:00 PM		
6:00 PM to 7:00 PM		
7:00 PM to 8:00 PM		
8:00 PM to 9:00 PM		
9:00 PM to 10:00 PM		
10:00 PM to 11:00 PM		
11:00 PM to Midnight		

Three Through Five Months

Day Two	Waking Time	Sleeping Time
Midnight to 1:00 AM		
1:00 AM to 2:00 AM		
2:00 AM to 3:00 AM		
3:00 AM to 4:00 AM		
4:00 AM to 5:00 AM		
5:00 AM to 6:00 AM		
6:00 AM to 7:00 AM		
7:00 AM to 8:00 AM		
8:00 AM to 9:00 AM		
9:00 AM to 10:00 AM		
10:00 AM to 11:00 AM		
11:00 AM to Noon		
Noon to 1:00 PM		
1:00 PM to 2:00 PM		
2:00 PM to 3:00 PM		
3:00 PM to 4:00 PM		
4:00 PM to 5:00 PM		
5:00 PM to 6:00 PM		
6:00 PM to 7:00 PM		
7:00 PM to 8:00 PM		
8:00 PM to 9:00 PM		
9:00 PM to 10:00 PM		
10:00 PM to 11:00 PM		
11:00 PM to Midnight		

Day Three	Waking Time	Sleeping Time
Midnight to 1:00 AM		
1:00 AM to 2:00 AM		
2:00 AM to 3:00 AM		
3:00 AM to 4:00 AM		
4:00 AM to 5:00 AM		
5:00 AM to 6:00 AM		
6:00 AM to 7:00 AM		
7:00 AM to 8:00 AM		
8:00 AM to 9:00 AM		
9:00 AM to 10:00 AM		
10:00 AM to 11:00 AM		
11:00 AM to Noon		
Noon to 1:00 PM		
1:00 PM to 2:00 PM		
2:00 PM to 3:00 PM		
3:00 PM to 4:00 PM		
4:00 PM to 5:00 PM		
5:00 PM to 6:00 PM		
6:00 PM to 7:00 PM		
7:00 PM to 8:00 PM		
8:00 PM to 9:00 PM		
9:00 PM to 10:00 PM		
10:00 PM to 11:00 PM		
11:00 PM to Midnight		

■ Day Four	Waking Time	Sleeping Time
Midnight to 1:00 AM		
1:00 AM to 2:00 AM		
2:00 AM to 3:00 AM		
3:00 AM to 4:00 AM		
4:00 AM to 5:00 AM		
5:00 AM to 6:00 AM		
6:00 AM to 7:00 AM		
7:00 AM to 8:00 AM		
8:00 AM to 9:00 AM		
9:00 AM to 10:00 AM		
10:00 AM to 11:00 AM		
11:00 AM to Noon		
Noon to 1:00 PM		
1:00 PM to 2:00 PM		
2:00 PM to 3:00 PM		
3:00 PM to 4:00 PM		
4:00 PM to 5:00 PM		
5:00 PM to 6:00 PM		
6:00 PM to 7:00 PM		
7:00 PM to 8:00 PM		
8:00 PM to 9:00 PM		
9:00 PM to 10:00 PM		
10:00 PM to 11:00 PM		
11:00 PM to Midnight		

■ Day Five	Waking Time	Sleeping Time
Midnight to 1:00 AM		
1:00 AM to 2:00 AM		
2:00 AM to 3:00 AM		
3:00 AM to 4:00 AM		
4:00 AM to 5:00 AM		
5:00 AM to 6:00 AM		
6:00 AM to 7:00 AM		
7:00 AM to 8:00 AM		
8:00 AM to 9:00 AM		
9:00 AM to 10:00 AM		
10:00 AM to 11:00 AM		
11:00 AM to Noon		
Noon to 1:00 PM		
1:00 PM to 2:00 PM		
2:00 PM to 3:00 PM		
3:00 PM to 4:00 PM		
4:00 PM to 5:00 PM		
5:00 PM to 6:00 PM		
6:00 PM to 7:00 PM		
7:00 PM to 8:00 PM		
8:00 PM to 9:00 PM		
9:00 PM to 10:00 PM		
10:00 PM to 11:00 PM		
11:00 PM to Midnight		

Three Through Five Months

■ Day Six	Waking Time	Sleeping Time
Midnight to 1:00 AM		
1:00 AM to 2:00 AM		
2:00 AM to 3:00 AM		
3:00 AM to 4:00 AM		
4:00 AM to 5:00 AM		
5:00 AM to 6:00 AM		
6:00 AM to 7:00 AM		
7:00 AM to 8:00 AM		
8:00 AM to 9:00 AM		
9:00 AM to 10:00 AM		
10:00 AM to 11:00 AM		
11:00 AM to Noon		
Noon to 1:00 PM		
1:00 PM to 2:00 PM		
2:00 PM to 3:00 PM		
3:00 PM to 4:00 PM		
4:00 PM to 5:00 PM		
5:00 PM to 6:00 PM		
6:00 PM to 7:00 PM		
7:00 PM to 8:00 PM		
8:00 PM to 9:00 PM		
9:00 PM to 10:00 PM		
10:00 PM to 11:00 PM		
11:00 PM to Midnight		

■ Day Seven	Waking Time	Sleeping Time
Midnight to 1:00 AM		
1:00 AM to 2:00 AM		
2:00 AM to 3:00 AM		
3:00 AM to 4:00 AM		
4:00 AM to 5:00 AM		
5:00 AM to 6:00 AM		
6:00 AM to 7:00 AM		
7:00 AM to 8:00 AM		
8:00 AM to 9:00 AM		
9:00 AM to 10:00 AM		
10:00 AM to 11:00 AM		
11:00 AM to Noon		
Noon to 1:00 PM		
1:00 PM to 2:00 PM		
2:00 PM to 3:00 PM		
3:00 PM to 4:00 PM		
4:00 PM to 5:00 PM		
5:00 PM to 6:00 PM		
6:00 PM to 7:00 PM		
7:00 PM to 8:00 PM		
8:00 PM to 9:00 PM		
9:00 PM to 10:00 PM		
10:00 PM to 11:00 PM		
11:00 PM to Midnight		

Six to Eight Months

✴ ● ✴ ● ✴ ● ✴ ● ✴ ● ✴ ● ✴ ● ✴ ● ✴ ● ✴ ● ✴ ● ✴ ● ✴ ● ✴ ● ✴ ●

SLEEP SIGNALS FROM SIX TO EIGHT MONTHS

Here you can write down what your baby does or how he acts just prior to sleeping. Don't forget that babies, even older ones, may not necessarily yawn or stretch or rub their eyes the way adults do.

For more information about sleep signals and sleep patterns from six to eight months, see pages 93 to 108.

Six to Eight Months

NOTE THE NAPS AND NIGHTS FROM SIX TO EIGHT MONTHS

Here are a week's worth of pages for you to track your baby's sleep. It's fine if you don't feel the need to track your baby's sleep for seven whole days. If you haven't already seen longer wakeful periods in the morning and evening, you probably will now. You may also notice another three-hour wakeful period between the morning and afternoon naps. If you are using the controlled-crying or fading technique to help your baby sleep at night, the sleep logs here can help you track your success.

   To use these logs, simply note the times that your baby sleeps: Write each of his wake times in the Waking Time column, and the start time of his naps and bedtime in the Sleeping Time column.

■ Day One	Waking Time	Sleeping Time
Midnight to 1:00 AM		
1:00 AM to 2:00 AM		
2:00 AM to 3:00 AM		
3:00 AM to 4:00 AM		
4:00 AM to 5:00 AM		
5:00 AM to 6:00 AM		
6:00 AM to 7:00 AM		
7:00 AM to 8:00 AM		
8:00 AM to 9:00 AM		
9:00 AM to 10:00 AM		
10:00 AM to 11:00 AM		
11:00 AM to Noon		
Noon to 1:00 PM		
1:00 PM to 2:00 PM		
2:00 PM to 3:00 PM		
3:00 PM to 4:00 PM		
4:00 PM to 5:00 PM		
5:00 PM to 6:00 PM		
6:00 PM to 7:00 PM		
7:00 PM to 8:00 PM		
8:00 PM to 9:00 PM		
9:00 PM to 10:00 PM		
10:00 PM to 11:00 PM		
11:00 PM to Midnight		

Six to Eight Months

	Waking Time	Sleeping Time		Waking Time	Sleeping Time
■ **Day Two**			■ **Day Three**		
Midnight to 1:00 AM			Midnight to 1:00 AM		
1:00 AM to 2:00 AM			1:00 AM to 2:00 AM		
2:00 AM to 3:00 AM			2:00 AM to 3:00 AM		
3:00 AM to 4:00 AM			3:00 AM to 4:00 AM		
4:00 AM to 5:00 AM			4:00 AM to 5:00 AM		
5:00 AM to 6:00 AM			5:00 AM to 6:00 AM		
6:00 AM to 7:00 AM			6:00 AM to 7:00 AM		
7:00 AM to 8:00 AM			7:00 AM to 8:00 AM		
8:00 AM to 9:00 AM			8:00 AM to 9:00 AM		
9:00 AM to 10:00 AM			9:00 AM to 10:00 AM		
10:00 AM to 11:00 AM			10:00 AM to 11:00 AM		
11:00 AM to Noon			11:00 AM to Noon		
Noon to 1:00 PM			Noon to 1:00 PM		
1:00 PM to 2:00 PM			1:00 PM to 2:00 PM		
2:00 PM to 3:00 PM			2:00 PM to 3:00 PM		
3:00 PM to 4:00 PM			3:00 PM to 4:00 PM		
4:00 PM to 5:00 PM			4:00 PM to 5:00 PM		
5:00 PM to 6:00 PM			5:00 PM to 6:00 PM		
6:00 PM to 7:00 PM			6:00 PM to 7:00 PM		
7:00 PM to 8:00 PM			7:00 PM to 8:00 PM		
8:00 PM to 9:00 PM			8:00 PM to 9:00 PM		
9:00 PM to 10:00 PM			9:00 PM to 10:00 PM		
10:00 PM to 11:00 PM			10:00 PM to 11:00 PM		
11:00 PM to Midnight			11:00 PM to Midnight		

Six to Eight Months

■ Day Four	Waking Time	Sleeping Time
Midnight to 1:00 AM		
1:00 AM to 2:00 AM		
2:00 AM to 3:00 AM		
3:00 AM to 4:00 AM		
4:00 AM to 5:00 AM		
5:00 AM to 6:00 AM		
6:00 AM to 7:00 AM		
7:00 AM to 8:00 AM		
8:00 AM to 9:00 AM		
9:00 AM to 10:00 AM		
10:00 AM to 11:00 AM		
11:00 AM to Noon		
Noon to 1:00 PM		
1:00 PM to 2:00 PM		
2:00 PM to 3:00 PM		
3:00 PM to 4:00 PM		
4:00 PM to 5:00 PM		
5:00 PM to 6:00 PM		
6:00 PM to 7:00 PM		
7:00 PM to 8:00 PM		
8:00 PM to 9:00 PM		
9:00 PM to 10:00 PM		
10:00 PM to 11:00 PM		
11:00 PM to Midnight		

■ Day Five	Waking Time	Sleeping Time
Midnight to 1:00 AM		
1:00 AM to 2:00 AM		
2:00 AM to 3:00 AM		
3:00 AM to 4:00 AM		
4:00 AM to 5:00 AM		
5:00 AM to 6:00 AM		
6:00 AM to 7:00 AM		
7:00 AM to 8:00 AM		
8:00 AM to 9:00 AM		
9:00 AM to 10:00 AM		
10:00 AM to 11:00 AM		
11:00 AM to Noon		
Noon to 1:00 PM		
1:00 PM to 2:00 PM		
2:00 PM to 3:00 PM		
3:00 PM to 4:00 PM		
4:00 PM to 5:00 PM		
5:00 PM to 6:00 PM		
6:00 PM to 7:00 PM		
7:00 PM to 8:00 PM		
8:00 PM to 9:00 PM		
9:00 PM to 10:00 PM		
10:00 PM to 11:00 PM		
11:00 PM to Midnight		

■ Day Six	Waking Time	Sleeping Time
Midnight to 1:00 AM		
1:00 AM to 2:00 AM		
2:00 AM to 3:00 AM		
3:00 AM to 4:00 AM		
4:00 AM to 5:00 AM		
5:00 AM to 6:00 AM		
6:00 AM to 7:00 AM		
7:00 AM to 8:00 AM		
8:00 AM to 9:00 AM		
9:00 AM to 10:00 AM		
10:00 AM to 11:00 AM		
11:00 AM to Noon		
Noon to 1:00 PM		
1:00 PM to 2:00 PM		
2:00 PM to 3:00 PM		
3:00 PM to 4:00 PM		
4:00 PM to 5:00 PM		
5:00 PM to 6:00 PM		
6:00 PM to 7:00 PM		
7:00 PM to 8:00 PM		
8:00 PM to 9:00 PM		
9:00 PM to 10:00 PM		
10:00 PM to 11:00 PM		
11:00 PM to Midnight		

■ Day Seven	Waking Time	Sleeping Time
Midnight to 1:00 AM		
1:00 AM to 2:00 AM		
2:00 AM to 3:00 AM		
3:00 AM to 4:00 AM		
4:00 AM to 5:00 AM		
5:00 AM to 6:00 AM		
6:00 AM to 7:00 AM		
7:00 AM to 8:00 AM		
8:00 AM to 9:00 AM		
9:00 AM to 10:00 AM		
10:00 AM to 11:00 AM		
11:00 AM to Noon		
Noon to 1:00 PM		
1:00 PM to 2:00 PM		
2:00 PM to 3:00 PM		
3:00 PM to 4:00 PM		
4:00 PM to 5:00 PM		
5:00 PM to 6:00 PM		
6:00 PM to 7:00 PM		
7:00 PM to 8:00 PM		
8:00 PM to 9:00 PM		
9:00 PM to 10:00 PM		
10:00 PM to 11:00 PM		
11:00 PM to Midnight		

Eight Months to One Year and Beyond

* ● * ● * ● * ● * ● * ● * ● * ● * ● * ● * ● * ● * ● * ● *

SLEEP SIGNALS FROM EIGHT MONTHS TO ONE YEAR AND BEYOND

Here you can write down what your baby does or how he acts just prior to sleeping. Don't forget that babies, even older ones, may not necessarily yawn or stretch or rub their eyes the way adults do.

For more information about sleep signals and sleep patterns from eight months to one year and beyond, see pages 108 to 114.

NOTE THE NAPS AND NIGHTS FROM EIGHT MONTHS TO ONE YEAR AND BEYOND

Here are a week's worth of pages for you to track your baby's sleep. It's fine if you don't feel the need to track it for seven whole days. By the end of the first year, nearly all babies will nap just twice daily, with wakeful periods that last either three hours or four and a half hours. It's still too early for most babies to give up their morning naps, but you may notice that this nap shortens. If you are teaching your baby sleep independence at night, the spaces here will help you keep track of your success.

To use these logs, simply note the times that your baby sleeps: Write each of his wake times in the Waking Time column, and the start time of his naps and bedtime in the Sleeping Time column.

▦ Day One	Waking Time	Sleeping Time
Midnight to 1:00 AM		
1:00 AM to 2:00 AM		
2:00 AM to 3:00 AM		
3:00 AM to 4:00 AM		
4:00 AM to 5:00 AM		
5:00 AM to 6:00 AM		
6:00 AM to 7:00 AM		
7:00 AM to 8:00 AM		
8:00 AM to 9:00 AM		
9:00 AM to 10:00 AM		
10:00 AM to 11:00 AM		
11:00 AM to Noon		
Noon to 1:00 PM		
1:00 PM to 2:00 PM		
2:00 PM to 3:00 PM		
3:00 PM to 4:00 PM		
4:00 PM to 5:00 PM		
5:00 PM to 6:00 PM		
6:00 PM to 7:00 PM		
7:00 PM to 8:00 PM		
8:00 PM to 9:00 PM		
9:00 PM to 10:00 PM		
10:00 PM to 11:00 PM		
11:00 PM to Midnight		

Eight Months to One Year and Beyond

■ Day Two	Waking Time	Sleeping Time	■ Day Three	Waking Time	Sleeping Time
Midnight to 1:00 AM			Midnight to 1:00 AM		
1:00 AM to 2:00 AM			1:00 AM to 2:00 AM		
2:00 AM to 3:00 AM			2:00 AM to 3:00 AM		
3:00 AM to 4:00 AM			3:00 AM to 4:00 AM		
4:00 AM to 5:00 AM			4:00 AM to 5:00 AM		
5:00 AM to 6:00 AM			5:00 AM to 6:00 AM		
6:00 AM to 7:00 AM			6:00 AM to 7:00 AM		
7:00 AM to 8:00 AM			7:00 AM to 8:00 AM		
8:00 AM to 9:00 AM			8:00 AM to 9:00 AM		
9:00 AM to 10:00 AM			9:00 AM to 10:00 AM		
10:00 AM to 11:00 AM			10:00 AM to 11:00 AM		
11:00 AM to Noon			11:00 AM to Noon		
Noon to 1:00 PM			Noon to 1:00 PM		
1:00 PM to 2:00 PM			1:00 PM to 2:00 PM		
2:00 PM to 3:00 PM			2:00 PM to 3:00 PM		
3:00 PM to 4:00 PM			3:00 PM to 4:00 PM		
4:00 PM to 5:00 PM			4:00 PM to 5:00 PM		
5:00 PM to 6:00 PM			5:00 PM to 6:00 PM		
6:00 PM to 7:00 PM			6:00 PM to 7:00 PM		
7:00 PM to 8:00 PM			7:00 PM to 8:00 PM		
8:00 PM to 9:00 PM			8:00 PM to 9:00 PM		
9:00 PM to 10:00 PM			9:00 PM to 10:00 PM		
10:00 PM to 11:00 PM			10:00 PM to 11:00 PM		
11:00 PM to Midnight			11:00 PM to Midnight		

Eight Months to One Year and Beyond

■ **Day Four**	Waking Time	Sleeping Time
Midnight to 1:00 AM		
1:00 AM to 2:00 AM		
2:00 AM to 3:00 AM		
3:00 AM to 4:00 AM		
4:00 AM to 5:00 AM		
5:00 AM to 6:00 AM		
6:00 AM to 7:00 AM		
7:00 AM to 8:00 AM		
8:00 AM to 9:00 AM		
9:00 AM to 10:00 AM		
10:00 AM to 11:00 AM		
11:00 AM to Noon		
Noon to 1:00 PM		
1:00 PM to 2:00 PM		
2:00 PM to 3:00 PM		
3:00 PM to 4:00 PM		
4:00 PM to 5:00 PM		
5:00 PM to 6:00 PM		
6:00 PM to 7:00 PM		
7:00 PM to 8:00 PM		
8:00 PM to 9:00 PM		
9:00 PM to 10:00 PM		
10:00 PM to 11:00 PM		
11:00 PM to Midnight		

■ **Day Five**	Waking Time	Sleeping Time
Midnight to 1:00 AM		
1:00 AM to 2:00 AM		
2:00 AM to 3:00 AM		
3:00 AM to 4:00 AM		
4:00 AM to 5:00 AM		
5:00 AM to 6:00 AM		
6:00 AM to 7:00 AM		
7:00 AM to 8:00 AM		
8:00 AM to 9:00 AM		
9:00 AM to 10:00 AM		
10:00 AM to 11:00 AM		
11:00 AM to Noon		
Noon to 1:00 PM		
1:00 PM to 2:00 PM		
2:00 PM to 3:00 PM		
3:00 PM to 4:00 PM		
4:00 PM to 5:00 PM		
5:00 PM to 6:00 PM		
6:00 PM to 7:00 PM		
7:00 PM to 8:00 PM		
8:00 PM to 9:00 PM		
9:00 PM to 10:00 PM		
10:00 PM to 11:00 PM		
11:00 PM to Midnight		

Eight Months to One Year and Beyond

■ **Day Six**	Waking Time	Sleeping Time
Midnight to 1:00 AM		
1:00 AM to 2:00 AM		
2:00 AM to 3:00 AM		
3:00 AM to 4:00 AM		
4:00 AM to 5:00 AM		
5:00 AM to 6:00 AM		
6:00 AM to 7:00 AM		
7:00 AM to 8:00 AM		
8:00 AM to 9:00 AM		
9:00 AM to 10:00 AM		
10:00 AM to 11:00 AM		
11:00 AM to Noon		
Noon to 1:00 PM		
1:00 PM to 2:00 PM		
2:00 PM to 3:00 PM		
3:00 PM to 4:00 PM		
4:00 PM to 5:00 PM		
5:00 PM to 6:00 PM		
6:00 PM to 7:00 PM		
7:00 PM to 8:00 PM		
8:00 PM to 9:00 PM		
9:00 PM to 10:00 PM		
10:00 PM to 11:00 PM		
11:00 PM to Midnight		

■ **Day Seven**	Waking Time	Sleeping Time
Midnight to 1:00 AM		
1:00 AM to 2:00 AM		
2:00 AM to 3:00 AM		
3:00 AM to 4:00 AM		
4:00 AM to 5:00 AM		
5:00 AM to 6:00 AM		
6:00 AM to 7:00 AM		
7:00 AM to 8:00 AM		
8:00 AM to 9:00 AM		
9:00 AM to 10:00 AM		
10:00 AM to 11:00 AM		
11:00 AM to Noon		
Noon to 1:00 PM		
1:00 PM to 2:00 PM		
2:00 PM to 3:00 PM		
3:00 PM to 4:00 PM		
4:00 PM to 5:00 PM		
5:00 PM to 6:00 PM		
6:00 PM to 7:00 PM		
7:00 PM to 8:00 PM		
8:00 PM to 9:00 PM		
9:00 PM to 10:00 PM		
10:00 PM to 11:00 PM		
11:00 PM to Midnight		

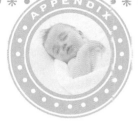

Special Circumstances

A bad cold, a trip across time zones, a painful episode of teething . . . sometimes it seems that life conspires to make a baby's good sleep go bad. Even parents who make sleep a high priority for their family will hit a few bumps now and then. This section shows you how to use your baby's rhythms to smooth over some of those bumps, or at least get you back on track quickly when life returns to normal. It also addresses the special concerns of parents who have multiple babies or babies who were born prematurely or at a low birthweight.

Illness

Illness can make your baby's sleepy signals more prominent. It can also make her window of alertness even shorter. For some babies who usually are able to stay awake for longer periods during the day, there may be a regression back to the 90-minute cycle. Go ahead and follow your baby's cues. Don't worry about the clock: Instead, watch her sleepy signals and allow her to sleep as much as she needs. Your baby will return to her normal sleep routine a few days after the illness is over.

When babies are ill, they often suffer from disrupted sleep, especially if the illness impairs their breathing. They may also require more physical contact and comforting than usual. Even if your baby has been sleeping independently up until now, you may want to bring your sick child into bed with you at night or even hold her in an upright position so breathing is easier. When the illness is over, you will probably need to reteach your baby to sleep alone. Generally, the teaching process is a little faster the second time around.

Teething

When a baby wakes up at night crying, people can be quick to assume "she must be teething." Teething is automatically offered as the culprit for night wakings, even when the wakings go on for days, weeks, or sometimes months. Yet the association between teething and night waking is greatly exaggerated, and very little data support it. The vast majority of night wakings in otherwise healthy and normally developing babies is caused by chronic sleep deprivation, not teething.

However, teething pain *does* sometimes occur at night, and the pain is real. Because the pain can occur well before the tooth is visible, it can take a while to learn when your baby is teething and when she is not. A good indicator is the type of cry she emits. Cries of pain are usually louder, higher pitched, and more insistent than the soft, whiny cries that babies often make when trying to return to sleep. If she isn't sick but is making a distressed sound, seems panicked, or is crying hard, she may well be cutting a tooth or two. Expect that she will need more comfort from you until the pain is over. You can also ask your pediatrician how to relieve teething pain. Once the pain is resolved (usually with the emergence of the tooth), know that you may have to reteach self-soothing techniques.

Jet Lag and Travel Across Time Zones

Babies don't know about time zones, but you can use their 90-minute cycles to reset their inner clocks when you're traveling across the country or around the world. I suggest using the 90-minute sleep cycle to keep the baby in a napping pattern until you have reached your destination and it is your baby's bedtime in the new time zone. For example, many flights to Europe depart in the late evening. When the plane lands, it is morning in the United States but late afternoon in the new time zone. Go ahead and use the 90-minute cycle to initiate sleep during the flight, but wake your baby up after 90 minutes. Then, 90 minutes following that awakening, put the baby to sleep again. Repeat this cycle as necessary, even after your arrival, until it's bedtime in your destination time zone. Then let the baby sleep as long as she likes. Parents using this method have told me that their babies adjust to jet lag more rapidly than they do.

By the way, I strongly caution against the use of diphenhydramine (Benadryl) or other medications to induce sleep in your infant while traveling. These drugs do not produce truly sound sleep, and sometimes they produce the opposite effect and make the baby hyperalert. And you probably know by now that depriving your baby of sleep in advance of a long flight won't lead to better sleep on the plane. That strategy can turn on you, producing a wild-eyed child who just can't settle down.

Daylight Saving Time

Parents dread springing forward and falling back! Be aware that it can take up to a week to adjust to the semiannual time changes. Although it's commonly believed that the Sunday on which the time change occurs is the most difficult, the brain actually struggles hardest on the following Monday. That's because the signals regarding darkness and bedtime are now mixed. In fact, there's a seasonal spike in traffic accidents on the Monday after the time change in spring when we lose an hour of sleep. Fall brings its own difficulties because babies don't usually take advantage of the opportunity to sleep in. Instead, they wake up an hour earlier, at least for a few days.

When the time changes, you and your child will need several days to adjust, so make your daily choices accordingly. Maybe this won't be the best time to tax your baby by running several errands in one day or to schedule important meetings at work, because you may not get as much sleep as usual. Also try to get as much natural sunlight as possible, to help your brain and your baby's brain resynchronize their internal functions.

Starting Child Care

When parents get the hang of the N.A.P.S. plan and see its benefits for their child, they become intent on making sure that the nanny, babysitter, grandparent, or child-care provider maintains the plan. Some parents worry that child-care centers, in particular, with their obligations to multiple children, will be unable to accommodate.

You may be pleasantly surprised, however. Most high-quality centers and caregivers understand the importance of infant and toddler sleep, even if they haven't heard of the 90-minute cycle specifically. I remember how difficult it was for me to leave my first child at a child-care center where no one had ever heard of the 90-minute rhythm. Because I didn't have much of a choice, I simply explained it to the head of the program as courteously as possible. I was worried that this very kind and very experienced woman, who had run her own child-care center for fifteen years and specialized in babies, was thinking "Uh-oh; another lunatic mother." But by the end of the first week, she said to me, "Boy, your daughter's like a *clock.*"

When you are choosing a child-care provider, look for someone who is caring and willing to listen to you. Speak candidly but respectfully about the 90-minute cycle, and see if the staff is willing to give it a try. If so, you can give the child-care workers a copy of the journal pages in the back of this book to help track your baby's naps. You may even make a few converts to the program! Also inquire about the center's nap policies. In some states, child-care centers are required by law to provide nap periods up to a specified age.

Twins and Other Multiples

I usually recommend going with the flow of a baby's sleep, letting a child sleep when she wants and for as long as she wants, but twins and other multiple babies constitute an exception. When you are trying to manage two, three, or more sets of sleep needs, it's okay to break the glass on the emergency box and use the 90-minute cycle to manipulate sleep schedules.

Parents of multiples can choose whether they want to have all their babies sleep at the same time (so the parents have some much-needed free time) or to have them awake separately (so as to spend one-on-one time with each child). Either way, you can control timing of naps by awakening the baby or babies 90 minutes before you want the next nap to occur. My children are not twins, but they were born only a year and a half apart, and for a few months their nap schedules were almost as complicated as those of multiples. I found I could use their 90-minute cycles to manage each day's challenges, but I made sure each child avoided sleep deprivation along the way.

Many multiples are born prematurely or at a low birthweight. Keep in mind that for a while, these babies may have a period of alertness shorter than 90 minutes. They may also have special feeding needs that require frequent wakings; if so, follow your doctor's advice.

Prematurity

Premature babies need even more sleep than babies who arrive on their due dates. Their window of alertness is usually shorter than 90 minutes; often, it's *much* shorter, with the baby able to stay awake for no longer than a few minutes after feeding. The baby requires this sleep to finish the brain development most babies undergo in utero. Just follow the baby's sleepy signals and help her sleep as much as possible. You will probably start to see the 90-minute cycle emerge when your baby is a few weeks past the date she was due to be born.

Be sure to follow your doctor's instructions about feeding the baby, even if you have to wake her up at regular intervals for feeding. Until you have the doctor's all-clear to allow longer sleep periods, keeping your premature baby nourished is your first priority.

Sleep Medications

Although some pediatricians recommend drugs like diphenhydramine (Benadryl) for common sleep problems, be careful about giving sleep medications to your child. There are some situations when a pediatrician will recommend sleep medications for a baby or young child, but it's not a good idea to rely on them as a way to solve garden-variety sleep difficulties. Most sleep agents fail to produce what specialists call physiological sleep, meaning that brainwaves don't have the same patterns that are produced by natural, undrugged sleep. Often, drug-induced sleep is shallow and unsatisfying. Rebound insomnia is another problem that occurs when a patient stops taking the drug, only to discover that she can't sleep without it. In addition, drugs like Benadryl can have a paradoxical effect on children, making them hyperalert. You have no way of knowing in advance whether your child will have this sort of response.

Sleep medications for children may be at their best when reserved for extreme cases with psychiatric or physical complications such as autism or in a temporary situation such as a hospitalization. Even then, their use should probably be the exception rather than the rule and should be limited to just a night or two, to break a cycle of sleep problems. If your doctor thinks your child should take a sleep medication, have a candid, thorough discussion with him or her about the benefits and disadvantages. Seek a second opinion if you need to.

When to Call the Doctor

At times sleep problems are caused by an underlying physical disorder.

Is Your Baby Caffeinated?

Few parents would pour out a shot of espresso for their little ones, but babies holding Sippy cups full of cola or eating chocolate cake with chocolate frosting are an increasingly common sight. Be aware of hidden sources of caffeine in common foods and medications. Chocolate, some sodas (check the label carefully—even orange soda and root beer can contain caffeine), some flavored waters, mocha ice cream, and of course tea, coffee, and coffee-based drinks and treats can all contain caffeine. Many over-the-counter cold medications contain stimulants and are another cause of mysteriously energized children (though note that cold medications should not be given to children under the age of two). My daughter is exceptionally sensitive to pseudoephedrine, a common decongestant. She'll stay awake for hours after taking it. My son, however, doesn't appear to be as sensitive to the drug.

Breastfeeding mothers often wonder if their coffee or chocolate habit is a cause of night wakings. Although the subject of breastfeeding, caffeine, and infant alertness is underinvestigated, most experts feel that a cup or two of coffee per day is unlikely to affect the baby's sleep. I suspect that most night wakings are caused by poor management of the 90-minute sleep rhythm rather than maternal caffeine intake However, if your baby follows the N.A.P.S. plan and is well rested but continues to struggle with wakefulness at night, you can certainly try eliminating caffeine from your diet for several days.

If your baby exhibits any of the following symptoms, contact your doctor:

Snoring that is not clearly caused by a cold or allergies. This may be an indication of a sleep-related breathing disorder similar to obstructive sleep apnea in adults. It's important to report this to your doctor even if your child breathes easily when awake.

Appearing to struggle with breathing while asleep, with loud breakthrough snorts or gasps. This is another symptom of a sleep-related breathing disorder. Your child may also do some sleep talking with this syndrome. The sleep talking by itself is not abnormal, and in many cases it goes away once the sleep/breathing difficulty is treated.

Frequent sleep attacks with loss of muscle tone. The sleep attacks may be accompanied by emotional excitement. The baby may be suffering from a seizure disorder or, in rare cases, narcolepsy.

Six or seven wakings each night after one year of age. It's unusual for babies to have this many wakings after the first year is over. It's a good idea to check things out with your doctor, just to rule out a medical cause for the wakings.

Index